T0384516

THE PSYCHOLOGY OF INNER PEACE

This book maps out the relationship between the discovery of heartfulness and the psychology of inner peace. It presents a rigorous psychological analysis of the underlying components of the psychology of inner peace and the role of innerness in addressing the nature of peace. Alternative theories are introduced that discuss the conceptualization of peace, and their merits are outlined in comparison to more mainstream psychological theories. The author highlights the inadequacies of mind-oriented theories on peace and demonstrates the concept of heartfulness to show how genuine peace can be achieved.

SAYYED MOHSEN FATEMI, Ph.D., is associate professor of psychology and chair of the Desk of North America at Ferdowsi University of Mashhad, Iran, and an adjunct faculty member in the Graduate Program in Psychology at York University, Canada. He is the recipient of the Ellen Langer International Mindfulness Award and runs psychotherapeutic and coaching programs for clinicians, practitioners, and businesses all over the world. He completed his postdoctoral studies in the department of psychology at Harvard University, where he has also served as a teaching fellow, an associate, and a fellow. In addition to teaching at Harvard, he has also taught for the department of psychology at the University of British Columbia, Western Washington University, University of Massachusetts in Boston, University of Toronto, York University, Ferdowsi University of Mashhad, Endicott College, and Boston Graduate School of Psychoanalysis.

THE PSYCHOLOGY
OF INNER PEACE

Discovering Heartfulness

SAYYED MOHSEN FATEMI, Ph.D.

Ferdowsi University of Mashhad

and

York University, Canada

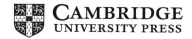

CAMBRIDGE
UNIVERSITY PRESS

CAMBRIDGE
UNIVERSITY PRESS

University Printing House, Cambridge CB2 8BS, United Kingdom

One Liberty Plaza, 20th Floor, New York, NY 10006, USA

477 Williamstown Road, Port Melbourne, VIC 3207, Australia

314–321, 3rd Floor, Plot 3, Splendor Forum, Jasola District Centre, New Delhi – 110025, India

79 Anson Road, #06–04/06, Singapore 079906

Cambridge University Press is part of the University of Cambridge.

It furthers the University's mission by disseminating knowledge in the pursuit of education, learning, and research at the highest international levels of excellence.

www.cambridge.org
Information on this title: www.cambridge.org/9781108489508
DOI: 10.1017/9781108784603

First published 2021

A catalogue record for this publication is available from the British Library.

Library of Congress Cataloging-in-Publication Data
NAMES: Fatemi, Sayyed Mohsen, 1964– author.
TITLE: The psychology of inner peace : discovering heartfulness / Sayyed Mohsen Fatemi,
Ferdowsi University and York University.
DESCRIPTION: New York, NY : Cambridge University Press, 2021. | Includes bibliographical references and index.
IDENTIFIERS: LCCN 2021002545 (print) | LCCN 2021002546 (ebook) | ISBN 9781108489508 (hardback) | ISBN 9781108747288 (paperback) | ISBN 9781108784603 (epub)
SUBJECTS: LCSH: Peace of mind. | Mindfulness (Psychology)
CLASSIFICATION: LCC BF637.P3 F37 2021 (print) | LCC BF637.P3 (ebook) | DDC 158.1–DC23
LC record available at https://lccn.loc.gov/2021002545
LC ebook record available at https://lccn.loc.gov/2021002546

ISBN 978-1-108-48950-8 Hardback
ISBN 978-1-108-74728-8 Paperback

Contents

v

Introduction

Writing this book comes at a time when the whole world is embroiled in COVID-19. The coronavirus has drastically influenced everyone and everything, from the routinized interaction of people in public places, such as restaurants, to higher education, marketing, and the business world. COVID-19 has perturbed the power of prediction, control, and decision making and has fueled anxiety, fear, and anger. The world is no longer what it used to be – a place where people could easily walk in the hallway, shake hands, and hug one another. The simplest modes of communication have turned out to be the most dangerous ones, with people avoiding touch and hugs in earnest.

Life has lost its familiar cycle these days, and there are no signs of vivacity and livelihood similar to the ones that existed prior to the coronavirus. The streets seem to be empty and avenues appear to be desolate and forlorn. Above all, feelings of fear and anxiety and the tremor of petrification resonate their certainty in the midst of an ambiguous world rife with stress and intolerance.

Speaking of peace has always been significantly vital for human civilization. Yet, this time unfolds a conspicuous urgency for creating a peace-oriented world. COVID-19 has highlighted a series of shifts in our seemingly taken-for-granted world; it has altered our epistemic axioms, our existential assumptions, and our unquestionably lived assumptions.

There have been numerous scholarly works on peace and its implementation. Their topics have focused on peace education, peace-building strategies, international peace, and so forth.

This book chooses a different approach and offers a new perspective. The book follows a number of goals and objectives: It presents the essentiality of peace in life for growth, development, well-being, wellness, and creativity. It offers a brief overview of the major outlooks that can reiterate the vitality of peace in our living. It demonstrates some of the closely knitted perspectives that propose and propound the ways and strategies that give rise to a peaceful world.

The distinctive features of the book that may espouse its salience in discussing the concept of peace coil around a string of interrelated issues: The defining characteristics of humanness may play a crucial role in achieving a sustainable, genuine, and authentic peace. The animalistic definition of human beings in their current forms may enable generative parlance on the conceptualization of peace and its ramifications but may not be able to thrive when it comes to establishing a pristine form of peace. Moreover, the exploration of ways and strategies to enliven peace in human communities needs to ultimately linger and visit human innerness in one way or another. This may pose the preponderance of a lively encounter with an influencing inner abode in human beings. Should there be no authenticity for the innerness of human beings, the peacekeeping and peace-building sources may appear to see their unsettling realm of claim.

Most important of all, this book offers a presentation of a new view on heart and heartfulness.

The Western world is first and foremost a world of calculation, rationality, linearity, analysis, reasoning, syllogism, and the mind. The foundations of this world propel its citizens to abide by the propositions that ultimately gain their sensibility within the mind-oriented framework. The mapping of this world is based on postulations that inextricably follow the mind-oriented framework.

The present book examines and presents the Western perspective on peace and then shifts to the Eastern perspective. Beginning with mainstream views of achieving peace at different levels, this book excavates their underlying guiding elements and argues for a new entry in the realm of psychology of peace. The book's arguments move toward a recondite analysis of peace structures within the human domain in the Western paradigm and then set out to underline a new paradigm known as heartfulness.

This book speaks of a new world different in shape and configuration, size and mode, nature and scope. The book posits a search within heart and heartfulness within a different paradigm that, albeit reconcilable with mind-driven human beings, calls for decomposing the taken-for-granted suppositions of the mind-driven world.

Although heart is brimming with polysemic implications in an unlimited repertoire of allusions and ascriptions, the book brings the concept of heartfulness beyond the frequently used discourse. In the heart of heartfulness, there lies the panacea of compassion, mercy, kindness, and benevolence. Heartfulness calls for exploring a new horizon in humanity, a horizon that has been less traveled in our era. This horizon looms in view of a flexible encounter with a new set of propositions that do not follow the well-taken-for-granted paradigms in mainstream psychology.

Understanding heartfulness may have some of its own challenges at face value since it might be linked with associations and emotionally ingrained responses that may have developed through the misrepresentation, distortion, and manipulation of transcendental, spiritual, and religious concepts. Extremist viewpoints on spirituality, religiosity, and mysticism may have left a tendency to mostly recall the noxious implications of the effects rather than examining the content and nature of the topic.

I need to mindfully express my gratitude to all those who had an impact on writing this book. My first thanks go to my son, Alisina, who was so encouraging and kind enough to read the book a few times while offering suggestions and insight. His attunement and support were great assets in upholding enthusiasm and fervor. My wife, Saqi, and my daughter, Sana, were patiently helpful during COVID-19 as they brought meaning and power to the pensive silence of reflexivity in the midst of turmoil and tension. My father, Mohammad, deserves special thanks, as his being a bibliophile has been very instrumental in composing great strides in thinking about thinking.

My late mother, Mahvash, to whom I owe an evergreen and eternal thankfulness, has been powerfully vital in espousing the seeds of heartfulness through her compassion and love.

I need to express my gratitude to David Repetto and Emily Watton at Cambridge University Press for their wonderful follow-up with the book project and their lively presence.

CHAPTER I

Peace

It is only with the heart that one can see rightly; what is essential is invisible to the eye.

Antoine de Saint-Exupéry

When discussing peace in relationships, whether interpersonal, intrapersonal, or international, peace is defined as a state of mind, a state of relationship, and a state of emotions, where tension, pandemonium, unrest, turmoil, chaos, and turbulence are replaced by tranquility, composure, equanimity, calmness, and serenity.

Some scholarly viewpoints have traced the roots of peace or lack of peace to the early relationships that a child may experience. This perspective maintains that right from the beginning of the birth (or even prior to the birth from a psychoanalytical point of view), a newborn is in need of receiving the gift and the pearl of connectedness. If the connection and the connectedness occur and the child experiences a welcoming position and a receiving attitude, he or she would experience security, trust, tranquility, and assurance as some of the main constituents of peace. Conversely, if the newborn encounters lack of understanding, lack of empathy, and lack of attunement, he or she would be lost in the barren land of despondency, mistrust, fear, anxiety, and doubts, which may serve as the major elements of creating tension.

What parents do verbally and nonverbally when dealing with a child in every moment of their interactions can espouse different psychological imprints in a child. Sensitive, responsive, and available parents pay attention to a child's needs, presence, and emotional wants and needs for connection and connectedness. As the beneficiaries of attentive, mindful, and meticulous attention and caring, careful strategies and approaches, children may experience the prerequisites of peace. On the other hand, parents who do not display and put into effect sensitive, available, and responsive attitudes and actions toward their children or use on-and-off, yes-and-no positions give rise to children who end up being anxious and avoidant in their lifestyle and communication patterns.

Thus, the preface of peace, from the attachment style perspective, may begin with early experiences of comfort, trust, support, understanding, empathy, sympathy, intersubjectivity, attunement, and love. The phenomenological experiences of tranquility would open up the doors to lived experiences that may facilitate the process of implementing peace in relationships.

Children who are raised by parents with paradoxical behaviors, condescending responses, invalidating approaches, and suppressive attitudes would most likely carry along the Zeigarnik effect throughout their lives – they can't be at peace with themselves and others since they have unmet needs that may consciously and unconsciously crop up in their interactions. A relationship's liveliness plays a significant role in one's well-being and wellness. The Center on the Developing Child (2020) at Harvard University indicates that children who have been neglected in a relationship may experience more drastically negative consequences and suffer more impairments than children who have been abused.

An attachment perspective on peace would have its main focus on the dynamics of early relationships, construction and manifestation of primordial relationships, the context of primary relationships and their implications for security and support, understanding and trust, insecurity and mistrust, and misunderstanding and fear (Ainsworth, 1982; Bowlby, 1973).

The turmoil of war is devastating, as is the turbulence of a tumultuous relationship. In his report to the World Health Organization (WHO) after World War II, Bowlby indicated that "the infant and young child should experience a warm, intimate and continuous relationship with his mother (or permanent mother substitute) in which both find satisfaction and enjoyment" (1954, p. 13).

The seed of peace is thus sowed in the early interactions of parents and children, which shape the psychological understanding of peace. Loss and separation, insensitivity, unresponsiveness, unavailability, coldness and indifference, and aggression and withdrawal in parent–child relationships would appear to be the impediments of experiencing an integrated, secure self.

A disintegrated, insecure self would be very much alien to the realm of peace. A child's frequent experiences of denial, suppression, repression, negligence, indifference, aggressiveness, loneliness, disconnectedness, despondency, despair, fear, anxiety, confusion, and mistrust would bring him or her a perturbable inner world with vulnerability.

In most of the literature on a secure sense of self, one may see the emphasis and analysis of scholars on the dynamics of early relationships between a child and his or her caregivers. Emotional distance between parents and children and lack of attunement have been considered as the major factors responsible for maladaptive emotions and psychological problems.

The emphasis here has been laid on the psychological needs. When emotional bids and psychological needs are neglected and ignored or have been aggressively dealt with, the result has appeared in unhealthy relationships in both intrapersonal and interpersonal domains.

Szyf, McGowan, and Meaney (2008, p. 160) highlight the importance of the emotional connection and says that major changes to our bodies can be made not just by chemicals and toxins, but also in the way the social world talks to the hardwired world.

On balance, psychological perspectives have explored and examined the roles of different needs in giving rise to a good sense of self and have built their theories based on the analytical demonstration of the given needs. In other words, numerous psychologists have discussed different needs and have considered some foundational needs as pivotal in espousing tension and unrest within the human psyche. Bowlby (1973) and other object relations theorists have underscored the need for relatedness as the cornerstone of peace and tranquility. Freud (1950) enunciated the maximization of pleasure and minimization of pain as crucial in affecting one's personality. In line with the pleasure principle, Dollard and Miller (1950), along with other scholars focusing on learning theories, have stressed the significance of pleasure and its contribution as a reinforcement in bringing calmness to one's personality. Phenomenological psychologists, including Rogers (1961), have discussed the need to maintain the stability and coherence of a person's conceptual system. Lack of coherence and incongruity have been considered major obstacles for achieving tranquility. Other psychologists, including Allport (1955) and Kohut (1971), have concentrated on the need for self-esteem enhancement.

Any of these psychological perspectives have proceeded with the assumptions that their identified needs within their system of thought can play a huge role in giving rise to human peace and that lack of satisfaction of those needs can play a major role in generating tension and turmoil within the human psyche. Psychopathology has been examined from the perspective of the imbalance among needs. Balance and coherence have been considered important aspects of one's well-being, health, and wellness.

It may be worthwhile to examine other implicitly influential factors that might address the possibility of peace in human life. This includes a hectic, intensive controversy over the analytical account of the mind and behavior and its diverse modalities that was characterized as the "hot approach versus cold approach" (e.g., see De Jaegher et al., 2010; Zajonc, 1984).

The hot perspective, which goes back to the 1950s and 1960s, was merely interested in the unconscious elements that produced certain types of performance. Thus, any performance, based on the hot perspective, was ultimately embedded within the unconscious interactive process with idiosyncratic emotional, cognitive, and behavioral categories. It was the realization of the hidden, clandestine, cryptic, and latently unconscious elements that contributed to the configuration of specific behavioral manifestation (e.g., see Zajonc, 1984).

An alternative perspective known as the cold approach was inspired by computer-oriented discoveries and focused on the cognitive interplay of the influencing factors of a performance. Focus on the impulsive, unconscious sedimentation of a behavior was here replaced with an interest in the analytical, computational, and serial processing of information and their implications for decision making in a performance. A search for the computational analysis of a performance and its original elements was encouraged in the cold perspective with the intention of identifying the systematic generative constituents of a performance (e.g., see De Jaegher et al., 2010; Rendel et al., 2011).

Both perspectives were challenged by critical approaches that indicated how each of the hot and cold outlooks overlooked some of the significant influential factors of a performance. The result was the combination of both perspectives into what was later called the "warm look" (e.g., see Sorrentino, 2003; Sorrentino & Higgins, 1986).

Dual process theories of social cognition examined two types of information processing that considered both hot and cold perspectives. One led to an effortful, reflective type of thinking, and the other one studied an automatic form of thinking, with both considering each of their implications for behavior and performance (Kruglanski & Orehek, 2007).

On the other hand, in his letter to Albert Einstein and in the body of his other writings, Freud adopts a deterministic view on human beings and proclaims the impossibility of peace; violence is ineluctably tied to human nature and human life (Freud, 1932, 1950, 1962).

Freud is not alone in proclaiming the impossibility of peace. The evolutionist camp to which he is adhering entails other thinkers who believe in the survival of the fittest through natural selection, and they comply with Freud's notion that peace is nothing but wishful thinking (Wilson, 1978). In one of his assertions, Freud (1918) says, "I have found little that is 'good' about human beings on the whole. In my experience most of them are trash."

Benito Mussolini was also on the same page when he said, "War is to man what maternity is to a woman. From a philosophical and doctrinal viewpoint, I do not believe in perpetual peace."

The war-stricken perspective is strongly embedded within a biological doctrine where aggression and violence are considered to be inextricably interwoven with the human system of life, human beings' general dispositions, and human beings' genetic predilections.

In compliance with Thomas Hobbes in reiterating that man is a wolf to man, Huntington posits that "it is human to hate" (1996, p. 130).

Adopting a political stance in explaining the human civilizations, Huntington turns down the possibility of peace, trust, and friendship and indicates that "cold peace, cold war, trade war, quasi war, uneasy peace, troubled relations, intense rivalry, competitive coexistence, arms races . . . are the most probable descriptions of relations between entities from different civilizations. Trust and friendship will be rare" (Huntington, 1996, p. 207).

The instinctual intensity of supremacy and power, the tyranny of biological determinism, and the strong desire to control may lead to the unquestionability of the impossible peace. The universality of war, the impossibility of peace, and the unquestionability of conflicts and turmoil are postulated in doctrines that ultimately deny the plausibility of implementing genuine peace in any form of relationships. On balance, one may discuss two paradoxical perspectives on peace: one that considers peace as an attainable goal and one that negates the possibility of establishing peace.

A Darwinian outlook has a focus on power and superiority. If existence is supposed to be run by the survival of the fittest and the key to success is to seek power and control, there would be an intrinsically emergent predilection toward hegemony. The ontological exegesis of domination in a Darwinian context would prescribe serious and strenuous attempts to secure power. The focus on domineering wealth and resources would give rise to a mentality of conflict, competitiveness, possessiveness, superiority, and polarization where you are either superior or inferior.

Exploring the nature of peace and its implications in sundry domains of human life including intrapersonal, interpersonal, and international relationships would ultimately lead us toward some vital questions, including the nature of humanness, the relationship between the inner world and the outer world, the defining components of human beings, the essence of peace in terms of its existential meaning, and other relevant questions and issues.

CHAPTER 2

The Western Approach toward Inner Peace

The mainstream Western perspective on peace may be reflected in sundry therapeutic schools of thought that focus on emotional, cognitive, and behavioral conflicts within human beings. The premise of these various viewpoints may have one common denominator: their interpretive angle on human beings as characterized in the material realm. In other words, the majority of these perspectives define human beings in the context of the material, tangible, and objective realities, considering no other dimensions. As human beings are embedded in the material realm, any curative attempt needs to be addressed, organized, and conceptualized within the material domain of human beings.

The movement in the 1940s and 1950s may be associated with a predilection toward a search in the unconscious world to find out what may cause the conflicts in the human world. The conflict among the id, ego, and superego; the emergence of the unconscious defense mechanism; the analysis of discontentment in civilizations; and the psychosexual developments in Freudian psychoanalysis may reveal one of many existing worldviews on human beings with a materialist concentration.

Freud's conceptualization of human beings is ultimately shaped by a system of thought wherein determinism supersedes human choices and the ideal possibility lies in an attainable management that, at its best, bridles human destructive instincts. Nonetheless, going beyond biological and psychological determinism is not conceivable. In discussing the nature of human beings, Freud (1918) says, "I have found little that is 'good' about human beings on the whole. In my experience most of them are trash." The conflicts between social and biological forces are inextricably tied to human nature in Freudian psychoanalysis. Such conflict in human inner forces may bring about destructiveness on both interpersonal and intrapersonal levels and thus may espouse complicated demolishing effects in the outside world, including war, genocide, massacre, and terrorism.

The psychoanalytical perspective is in pursuit of understanding the mystery behind the unconscious forces and their motivating power in shaping and changing realities. Freud's attempt is to explain the mechanism of destructiveness in the human realm through a deep search within the human psyche and its surreptitious and clandestine sources in creating conflicts and pandemonium. In his letter to Albert Einstein, Freud writes,

> Conflicts of interest between man and man are resolved, in principle, by the recourse to violence. It is the same in the animal kingdom, from which man cannot claim exclusion; nevertheless, men are also prone to conflicts of opinion, touching, on occasion, the loftiest peaks of abstract thought, which seem to call for settlement by quite another method. This refinement is, however, a late development. To start with, group force was the factor which, in small communities, decided points of ownership and the question which man's will was to prevail. Very soon physical force was implemented, then replaced, by the use of various adjuncts; he proved the victor whose weapon was the better, or handled the more skillfully. Now, for the first time, with the coming of weapons, superior brains began to oust brute force, but the object of the conflict remained the same: one party was to be constrained, by the injury done him or impairment of his strength, to retract a claim or a refusal. This end is most effectively gained when the opponent is definitely put out of action – in other words, is killed. This procedure has two advantages: the enemy cannot renew hostilities, and, secondly, his fate deters others from following his example. Moreover, the slaughter of a foe gratifies an instinctive craving.... However, another consideration may be set off against this will to kill: the possibility of using an enemy for servile tasks if his spirit be broken and his life spared. Here violence finds an outlet not in slaughter but in subjugation. Hence springs the practice of giving quarter; but the victor, having from now on to reckon with the craving for revenge that rankles in his victim, forfeits to some extent his personal security.

The psychoanalytical perspective led by Freud does not conceive of any reality except the materially embedded representations that are of an objective, visible, and tangible quiddity. For Freud, God is merely a demonstration of a longing for a protective father figure who provides comfort and security for people embroiled in anxiety and fear. In his book *The Future of an Illusion*, Freud dismisses the truth of God and considers it a collective neurosis.

Along with the psychoanalytical perspective on human nature and its emphasis on the materialistic essence of human beings, similar emergent viewpoints on human nature in the Western world have underlined the search for human peace in connection with the relationships between thoughts, feelings, and behaviors and their synchronicity and congruence.

Cognitive behavioral therapy (CBT), for instance, examines how unquestionably accepted beliefs may give rise to numerous signs of anxiety and conflict in one's behavior and teaches clients to debate their systems of beliefs. Various kinds of CBT, including the techniques of Goldfried and Davison (1976), Maultsby (1975), Meichenbaum (1977), and Rimm and Masters (1979), examine the possibility of removing tension from the human mind.

Simultaneously, social psychologists and researchers who have studied performance indicated that positive messages, enhancement of conversations among team members between and during plays, expression of emotions, and team cohesion are positively correlated with positive performance (see Dale & Wrisberg, 1996; DiBerardinis et al., 1983; Lausic et al., 2009).

Likewise, in the psychopharmaceutical world, the questions revolve around what brings about tranquility and the mechanisms that may impede the process of achieving a calm brain. Neurotransmitters are explored and examined in terms of their dynamics and interactions in a synaptic neural network to demonstrate turbulence and tumult in a brain on fire.

The medical world, inspired by the medical and biological model, has sharpened its focus mainly on discovering the physical realm of the neural networks to unearth the secrets that may lead to the possibility of having access to a peaceful brain. Disruptions in the neurotransmitters' activities, genetic components, and heredity, along with damage to different parts of the brain, have been considered as responsible for giving rise to a brain on fire.

In the meantime, violence has been examined in Western psychological perspectives with a focus on both internal and external factors. Internal factors have focused on age, gender, personality traits, and hostile cognitive biases (e.g., see Archer, 2000; Dill et al., 1997; Paulhus & Williams, 2002; Tremblay, 2000). External factors have explored the roles of weapons, alcohol, the media, and unpleasant events along with their relevant frustration in advancing the cycle and scope of tension and violence (e.g., see Anderson et al., 2010; Berkowitz, 1989; Gailliot & Baumeister, 2007; Hemenway, Vriniotis, & Miller, 2006; Subra et al., 2010).

One important point to note here is that within the expansive and immensely operable schools of thought approaching human dynamics in the mainstream Western perspective, there is an underlying infrastructure that ultimately represents humans in terms of their materialistic nature. This pervasive perspective's assumptions and axioms define human beings in terms of their physical, material, physiological, and neurological aspects.

The psychological facets are presented in the body of the material components; that is, the psychological pieces are embedded within the material and neurological aspects.

Moreover, the postulations presenting materialistic hermeneutics of humans have been considerably challenged within the Western system. In challenging the materialistic viewpoint on explaining human dynamics, Spariosu (2004, 94) indicates that

> [m]ost mainstream scientists are no more ready than Wilson to give up the ideology of evolutionary progress and success that has supposedly served them so well. Of course, in their rare self-reflective moments these scientists see themselves, at least in print, as disinterested, selfless seekers and servers of objective knowledge and truth. Indeed, they see themselves as worshippers in the "Temple of Science" as Albert Einstein very aptly (and with no trace of irony or self-irony) puts it. In practice, however, those claiming to be in possession of the truth, or at least of parts of it, are stern, Cerberian gatekeepers to this new temple, and will exact a high price to let noninitiates and neophytes in.

In line with a critique of the materialist view of human beings, Beauregard and O'Leary (2007, xv) also indicate that

> [m]aterialism is apparently unable to answer key questions about the nature of being human and has little prospect of ever answering them ineligibly. It has also convinced millions of people that they should not seek to develop their spiritual nature because they have none.

Ernest Becker voiced his critique against the reductionism of humanness and described reliance on the scientific method for understanding human beings as self-defeating (1971, 1973).

Comporting with a critique of the materialist perspective on humanness, Spariosu (2004, 5) states,

> Our global pundits, whether on the right or the left, seem to connect human progress primarily with material development. Most worldwide statistics and indicators are economic in nature, measuring human happiness by what an individual or a social group has, rather than by what they are. Thus, we have presently divided the world into "developed," "underdeveloped," and "developing" societies. But if we truly wish to change our global paradigms, then we need to change the focus of our worldwide efforts from social and economic development to human self-development. From the standpoint of the latter, there are no developed or underdeveloped societies, but only developing ones. It is this kind of development that in the end will help us solve our practical problems, including world hunger, poverty, and violence, and will turn the earth into a welcoming and nurturing home for all of its inhabitants, human and nonhuman.

From yet a different intellectual position, Roger Scruton (2009) also questions the sovereignty of modern biotechnological reductionism when he discusses the implications of Milton's poetry:

> Milton's allegory is not just a portrait of our kind; it is an invitation to kindness. It shows us what we are, and what we must live up to. Take away religion, however; take away philosophy, take away the higher aims of art, and you deprive ordinary people of the ways in which they can represent their apartness. Human nature, once something to live up to, becomes something to live down to instead. Biological reductionism nurtures this "living down," which is why people so readily fall for it. It makes cynicism respectable and degeneracy chic. It abolishes our kind; and with it our kindness. (107)

In line with his critique of the utilitarian epistemology of Western mainstream scientific discourse, Spariosu (2004) highlights the significance of an open approach to the possibility of exploring non-Western intercultural perspectives:

> Within the globality of our planet, there may be – or one may imagine – many different worlds that are not primarily driven by the utilitarian, free market logic described by Western-style, neoliberal, post-Marxist, and postmodernist theorists. Therefore, it is our task not only to identify or imagine such worlds, but also to work collectively toward their (re-) emergence as alternatives to the current ones, which have largely proven to be unsustainable. (45)

Critiquing mainstream psychology's approach toward humanness and discussing the prevalence of different limiting paradigms in defining the nature of human beings (including the formalistic paradigms of natural science, psychoanalysis, behaviorism, cognitive science, and neuroscience,) Schneider (2011) indicates that

> I believe that psychology should now be reset on its rightful base in existence. It is high time that psychology recognized what the great poets and thinkers the world over have recognized for centuries – that the main problem of the human being is the paradoxical problem: that we are both angels and food for worms; that we are suspended between constrictive and expansive worlds, and that we are both exhilarated and stupefied by this tension. The role this leaves for humanistic psychology is the role that William James so deftly set for it back in 1902. That was the year James wrote *Varieties of Religious Experience* and called for a radically empirical, experientially informed inquiry into the human being's engagement with the world (Taylor, 2010). I also believe that humanistic psychology's role today is commensurate with the existential-phenomenological-spiritual tradition of successors to James (see Mendelowitz & Kim, 2010), exemplified

by Paul Tillich (1952), Martin Buber (1970), Rollo May (1981), R.D. Laing (1969), Ernest Becker (1973), and many others who called for a new "whole bodied" experience of inquiry and life.

Furthermore, some scholarship has questioned the essence and substance of research programs in humanities and science as well as the funding of projects that may seemingly take place for the sake of peace and wellness. Pinxten (2009, 192) elaborates this and indicates that

> [i]n a very general way I hold that scientific research is embedded in the sociopolitical and the cultural context of the West. The sociopolitical embeddedness implies that funding, promotion chances and even freedom of research will be codetermined by the political context of the researcher to a smaller or larger extent. In the case of the humanities this point has been illustrated by such volumes as Chomsky (1996) and Nader (2000), which show how the development of the Humanities in the 1960s and 1970s of the past century were influenced and sometimes curtailed by the military and political powers of the USA. In a similar vein, the explicit offer of research jobs by the CIA (in the USA) and by M15 (in the UK) from 2006 on through advertisements in the major anthropological journals gave rise to a debate in the discipline; it is clear that the freedom of research is not guaranteed in these circumstances, knowing that already in the past anthropological results have been (ab)used in warfare, without the awareness or consent of the researchers (Houtman 2006).

On the other hand, scholars have extensively discussed Western humanism as a complex historical, sociopolitical, philosophical, and religious phenomenon whereby the sovereignty and centrality of human values in producing methods, practices, and policies in a specific society were given prominence over any other worldview. They have explored and revealed the sundry historical manifestations of humanism in different literary, philosophical, and cultural contexts, and in different parts of the world, although particularly in Europe. Renaissance humanism and Italian humanism have been explored in the body of such historical excavation, whereas the Greek, British, and German forms have been discussed in line with an interest in the periodic emergence of humanism in different eras.

Additionally, different forms of emphasis have emerged in each of these historic manifestations: For instance, German humanism tended toward ethnocentrism, whereas another notable humanist trend sought to dissociate itself from the church. The political, social, and philosophical facets of humanism have also been understood in terms of the antecedent, precipitating factors that gave rise to their emergence, with the intention of challenging the social status quo. In this regard, pedagogical humanistic trends have both deconstructed traditional layers of education and attempted to reconstruct new lines of thinking and learning.

The deepening semiotics of humanism has also challenged a number of traditional religious ideas, values, and doctrines and has resorted, instead, to secular avenues of social or intellectual engagements that it often offered as a panacea for lost and confused human beings.

To certain types of humanism, detachment from heavenly discourses and the adoption of secular modes of thinking appeared to promise the happiness and welfare that seemed to burgeon in the ideal illustration of humanism's values. Overall, many humanistic trends advanced sweeping claims for man's liberation and emancipation from everything, including God. They shifted the focus from man's ascension to heaven to his establishment on earth, away from any dependency on transcendental sources.

In addressing the content and subject matter of psychology as a discipline that needs to focus on human nature and explore the what and why of humanness in a profoundly foundational approach, Fisher (2004, xx) indicates that

> [b]y now, with psychology having been established as a rigorous empirical discipline, most psychologists no longer accept the "control and predict" definition and no longer cite logical positivism and related philosophical foundations, but often do count on accepted experimental procedures and statistical analysis as adequate to continue building a body of knowledge. Psychology textbooks most often define psychology as the study of human and animal behavior.

Carl Rogers discussed an example in psychology that leaves a Christian view of God, sin, and reconciliation to God and shifts to the human's purpose as being to actualize one's innate person through unconditional acceptance. Relation to another being (God in particular) is secondary to the goal of finding one's true self apart from the evaluations of others. Maybe God or others can have a place, but the goal is now focused on the self. Of course, there are milder views, such as that of Abraham Maslow, where belongingness has a place midway on the hierarchy while the apex is still focused on self-actualization and not on anything divine.

When discussing materialism here, the focus is on the materialist ontology where human being is reduced to matter. On the other hand, this does not tend to overgeneralize the materialist ontology to all Western psychological schools of thought, but only to the ones seeking the truth merely in the five senses, the visible, and the manifest world.

In defense of the materialist ontology, Russell (1903) rejects any possibility of existence and sensibility beyond the material world and iterates that

> [m]an is the product of causes which had no prevision of the end they were achieving; that his origin, his growth, his hopes and fears, his loves and his beliefs are but the outcome of accidental collocations of atoms; that no fire, no heroism, no intensity of thought and feeling, can preserve an individual life beyond the grave; that all the labours of the ages, all the devotion, all the inspiration, all the noonday brightness of human genius, are destined to extinction in the vast death of the solar system, and that the whole temple of Man's achievement must inevitably be buried beneath the debris of a universe in ruins − all these things, if not quite beyond dispute, are yet so nearly certain, that no philosophy which rejects them can hope to stand.

Expanding on his materialist ontology, Russell (1903) turns down the meaningfulness of any immaterial experience and says, "We can make no distinction between the man who eats little and sees heaven and the man who drinks much and sees snakes. Each is in an abnormal physical condition, and therefore has abnormal perceptions."

For materialism, humanness is characterized in physicality, and there would be no immaterial components for human beings. Armstrong (1968, 11) indicates that "[f]or a Materialist, a man is a physical object, distinguished from other physical objects only by the special complexity of his physical organization." In a later example of a materialist ontology, Wilson (1998, 291) describes human beings as "extremely complicated machines" and presents "consilience," wherein the central idea emphasizes the material nature of human beings.

In addition to the materialist ontology, the mainstream Western perspective on human nature vitalizes the necessity of objectivism, naturalism, scientism, universality, and a discourse of supremacy. The overall perspective excludes any possibility of sensibility outside the parameters of an objective discourse where verification, experimentation, quantification, refutability, replication, and reductionism highlight their prominence.

Human nature is thus inextricably tied to a cynosure of material causes within biological systems that are ultimately subsumed under an evolutionary pattern of the Darwinian paradigm. In understanding human nature within the evolutionary paradigm, one needs to inevitably postulate a plethora of propositions that continue to operate on the strength of reiterating that human nature is understandable in a fully material world, and there would be no meaning, purpose, design, goal, or direction outside the material world.

Through acquiring scientific knowledge and its specifically defined methodology, we can come to realize human nature in a systematic, accumulative manner. As the laws of physics help us understand the mysteries of matter and particles, we can formulate generalizable laws that help us decipher the secrets of human nature.

Apart from the critiques that have followed the materialistic perspective on human nature away from an investigation into the veracity of the axioms that have been taken for granted by the materialism camp, the generation of a discourse of supremacy is noteworthy here.

I have already demonstrated that such a discourse lies "on the legitimacy of the perspective of the knower, namely the expert who, at the center of discourse of power, could collect and analyze the data and then embark on generalizing the information for the sake of generative theories" (Fatemi, 2016).

The result of such supremacy has nurtured the promotion of an imperialist view on human nature where the hegemony of the expert's perspective is entitled to draw the lines of plausibility and prescribe epistemic, ethical, ontological, and teleological movements. Peace, therefore, needs to be obtained and granted by virtue of a methodology and a systematization that rely on the scientific discourse of the pervasive paradigm.

A subtle point to consider here is understanding the differences between a psychological explanation of peace that can occur in view of differing perspectives, albeit materialist or immaterialist, and the leading perspective from which the realization and implementation of peace are proposed and propounded in line with their exegesis of human nature.

In other words, if the leading perspective on peace is inspired by a worldview where human beings are solely defined in terms of their biological configuration and their inner world is characterized through the interplay of a biological, physiological, and neurological system, then the psychology of inner peace can ultimately envision an organismic synergy where the balance of the physicality of the aforementioned components – namely, the biological, physiological, and neurological facets – transpire. Conversely, if human nature is existentially expanded and goes beyond the physicality of the sphere of the appearance of human beings, then alternative modes of inquiry can make sense.

The abovementioned clarification is of vital importance with respect to the upcoming points since it facilitates the process of coming to know how different epistemological and ontological paradigms may espouse two entirely different lines of direction. In one perspective, the *self* is embodied in the physicality of the dynamics of neurons and the brain; thus, there is no innerness or inwardness beyond the perceptibility of the manifest features of life and their atomic aggregation in a collected system of operation. In another perspective, the innerness occupies a special status: It brings its own merit and worth; it propounds a transcendental inwardness. This second view's interpretation of the self exceeds Wilsonian consilience and supersedes Darwinian social degeneration.

The mainstream Western paradigm has long been preoccupied with a reductionist attempt to provide a linear analysis of human dynamics in the context of the so-called scientific outlook. This scientific outlook has been mainly run in the body of traditional empiricism and has circumscribed the scope of inquiries into hallmarks that do not allow investigations that lie outside the margins of the pre-identified scientism.

In elaborating the complexity of well-being, health, wellness, and peace and going beyond the reductionism in mainstream psychology, Schneider (2018) critiques the foundational elements of the psychological approach and indicates that

> [t]here is a reason that many of the most twisted and destructive people on this planet are not seen as "mental patients." They tend to be ordinary or even celebrated individuals – and their brains are as "normal" as the rest of us. Does this not tell us something glaring about the inadequacy of our current diagnostic system, as well as the culture out of which it arises? We have no language for the malady that both supersedes and in many cases fuels the diagnostic categories we conventionally term psychiatric illnesses, and our reduction of them to brain abnormalities almost entirely blinds us to their deeper cause. This cause is overridingly environmental and the product not of sickness but of unaddressed, unacknowledged fear – which leads individuals – as well as societies – to become rigid, narrow, and destructive. (p. 100)

Schneider broadens the scope of understanding tension and peace beyond the *DSM* (American Psychiatric Association, 2000) diagnosis and states,

> But even more importantly – and unlike conventional diagnoses – the state is as applicable to the rich and powerful (who have arguably done the most humanitarian damage) as it is to the poor and destitute, and to the societal as well as to the individual. (Schneider, 2018, p. 102)

In revisiting the certitude of the mainstream psychological research, Langer (2005) indicates that

> [s]cience, which prides itself on its objectivity, usually hides its choices from us even as it reports its findings. Many design choices that go into even our most rigorous scientific studies affect their outcomes. Greater awareness of these choices would make the findings less absolute and more useful to us.

In fact, scientific research is reported in journals as probability statements, although textbooks and popular magazines often report the same results as absolute facts. This change is done to make the science easier for the non-scientists to understand. But what it does, instead, is deceive us by promoting an illusion of stability. That illusion is fostered by taking people out of the equation – what choices the researcher made in sitting up the experiment, on whom it was tested, and under what circumstances. (p. 106)

If human nature is explicated in a merely mechanical, machine-oriented, linear, and material context, then questions of meaning, design, direction, and goals are ineluctably proliferated in the same context, albeit advanced in terms of level and quality. The possibility of understanding and achieving inner peace will be bound by the doctrine that is surrounded by its own intrinsic contingencies, namely, materialism, objectivism, perceptibility, physicality, reductionism, linearity, and materialistic causality.

The alleged objectivity in the scientific discourse on humanity has been long subjected to rigorous critique. This so-called objectivity, Kierkegaard argues, cannot let us explore the nature of innerness. Kierkegaard's challenge of Hegelian rationality and the objectivity of Hegelians such as Martensen calls for revamping the foundations of knowing and knowledge as it reveals the circumscribing pillars of objectivity in the discourse of rationality. In *Concluding Unscientific Postscript*, Kierkegaard's (1992) pseudonymous Johannes Climacus argues that objectivity cannot give rise to inwardness.

Kierkegaard claims that just as lack of objective truth can lead to madness, the "absence of inwardness is madness" too. Climacus illustrates a patient who has just escaped from a mental hospital and is worried about being recognized. He is worried that right after recognition, he will be sent back to the hospital, so he thinks to himself,

> "What you need to do, then, is to convince everyone completely, by the objective truth of what you say, that all is well as far as your sanity is concerned." As he is walking along and pondering this, he sees a skittle ball lying on the ground. He picks it up and puts it in the tail of his coat. At every step he takes, this ball bumps him, if you please, on his bottom, and every time it bumps him he says, "Boom! The earth is round!" He arrives in the capital city and immediately visits one of his friends. He wants to convince him that he is not crazy and therefore walks back and forth, saying continually "Boom! The earth is round!" (Kierkegaard, 1992, p. 195)

Kierkegaard (1992) also argues that

> objectively the emphasis is on what is said; subjectively the emphasis is on how it is said.... But this is not to be understood as manner, modulation of

voice, oral delivery, etc., but it is to be understood as the relation of the existing person, in his very existence, to what is said. Objectively, the question is only about categories of thought; subjectively, about inwardness.... Only in subjectivity is there decision, whereas wanting to become objective is untruth. The passion of the infinite, not its content, is the deciding factor, for its content is precisely itself. In this way the subjective "how" and subjectivity are the truth. (p. 203)

Kierkegaard laments against the selflessness of the modern age and deplores the impediments that get in the way of people's actualization of the self. Kierkegaard argues that dissipation of the self contributes to our despair and despondency, as it hampers our being fully human.

Contrary to the atheistic existentialism of Sartre and Camus, Kierkegaard considers renaissance of the self through a connection to the spirit as he elucidates that

a human being is a spirit. But what is spirit? Spirit is the self. But what is the self? The self is a relation that relates itself to itself or is the relation's relating itself to itself in the relation; the self is not the relation but is the relation's relating itself to itself. A human being is a synthesis of the infinite and the finite, of the temporal and the eternal, of freedom and necessity, in short, a synthesis. A synthesis is a relation between two. Considered in this way, a human being is still not a self. (Kierkegaard, 1989, p. 43)

In critiquing mainstream psychology and its predilections on taxonomy, categorizations, and classifications, Sundararajan (2020) argues that the prescriptive categorizations impose a reductionist and parochial outlook that impedes the process of celebrating humaneness in a broad cultural sphere.

This may also lead to a clandestine form of alienation and estrangement from others who may supposedly stand outside the cycle of the taken-for-granted categories.

Furthermore, Sundararajan (2020) indicates how the hegemony of mainstream psychology's mass production of knowledge within its own paradigm may bring us a perfunctory relationship to both you and me without an authentic quest for creating values that can espouse a genuine sense of togetherness. Her arguments demonstrate that the hegemony of abstract categorization prevents us from engaging with the culturally different Other as persons.

Sundararajan's (2020) critique of the Western-oriented taxonomy may highlight the significance of Kierkegaard's play of passion and practice. Kierkegaard disdains the viewpoint on philosophy that is merely engaged in the abstract conversations of the past. In his pseudonymous book *either/or*, Kierkegaard (1959) demonstrates how his philosophy is not in pursuit of the same principles of his contemporary philosophers and states,

> The philosopher says, "That's the way it has been hitherto." I ask, "what am I to do if I don't want to become a philosopher?" For if I want to do that, I see clearly enough that I, like the other philosophers, shall soon get to the point of mediating the past.... There is no answer to my questions of what I ought to do, for if I was the most gifted philosophical mind that ever lived in the world, there must be one more thing I have to do besides sitting and contemplating the past. (pp. 171, 175)

Russellian, Wilsonian, and Darwinian pedagogy of peace would not lead to any epiphanic, insightful, or inspirational discovery of an ontological sensibility of an inner peace. In fact, there is no innerness beyond the exterior and exteriorized manifestation of the material visibility of humans. The psychological realm of investigation will not recognize the broader possibility of probing the unknown beyond the mastery of an objective viewpoint and its hallmarks.

Darwinian evolutionary theory, Wilsonian biological theory of culture and society in the form of sociobiology, and Russell's materialistic view of human existence leave no room for the presence of any soul, any spirit, any you, or any innerness. There is merely the visible "you" in the physical world, and you just need to decipher the secrets to move on and gain your superiority to not be defeated and overrun by the others. As Wilson (1998, p. 76) puts it, "In war – and Nature is a battlefield, make no mistake – one needs secret codes." Here, one must emphasize how inner peace itself may be subjected to pandemonium and tension if the source of peace is to be sought in the material world.

Teo (2005) presents a wide variety of examples and evidence to corroborate how mainstream psychology has contributed to racism, oppression, crime, suffering, and injustice. He demonstrates how the production of knowledge in mainstream psychology has not necessarily led to the promotion of public good and has not been of service to humanness and peace. In elucidating some of these examples, he elaborates that

> [o]n the background of scientific racism, it was not sufficient to state problems, but also to provide arguments and seemingly logical and empirical justifications for these negative assessments. Gobineau (1854–1966) had learned that native women in certain parts of Oceania who had become mothers by Europeans could no longer become pregnant by their native men. Based on this "evidence" Gobineau (1816–1882) concluded that civilizations that were based on racially distinct groups should never come

together. Broca (1864) cited a medical argument to the effect that the large African penis coincided with the size of the African vagina. This meant that a white man could have sex with an African woman because intercourse would be easy and without any inconveniences for the African woman. However, sex between an African man and a white woman would make sex painful for the white woman. In addition, such a union often not lead to reproduction and thus should be avoided. (p. 174)

In line with delineating the problems with mainstream psychology in addressing authentic tranquility for human beings, Nelson and Prilleltensky (2005) highlight "chilling" quotes from Albee (1981):

We face the possibility of racial admixture here that is infinitely worse than that favoured by any European country today, for we are incorporating the Negro into our racial stock while all of Europe is comparatively free from this taint ... the decline of American intelligence will be more rapid ... owing to the presence of the Negro (Brigham [Princeton psychologist], 1923). [Massive sterilization] is a practical, merciful and inevitable solution of the whole problem, and can be applied to an ever widening circle of social discards, beginning always with the criminal, the diseased, and the insane and extending gradually to types which may be called weaklings rather than defectives and perhaps ultimately to worthless race types (Grant [New York Zoological Society], 1919). (Nelson and Prilleltensky 2005, p. 8)

Expanding the critique on mainstream psychology in dealing with human challenges and social problems, Nelson and Prilleltensky (2005) indicate that

[a]s an example, the field of psychology had created intelligence testing in the UK (Francis Galton) and France (Alfred Binet) and IQ tests were imported to and refined in the US during this period. Galton and other psychologists in the area of intelligence testing were proponents of Social Darwinism (Albee, 1996a), which took Darwin's concepts of natural selection and survival of the fittest and applied them to human beings and intelligence. IQ was viewed as an innate quality of individuals, and people with low IQ scores were seen as inferior and unworthy, people who should be "weeded out" of society because they weakened the genetic stock. The eugenics movement, which was prominent in the 1920s, used the philosophy of Social Darwinism to advocate for the separation of the "feeble-minded" from the rest of society into institutions, sterilization of people with low IQ, and restrictions on the immigration of people deemed to be inferior (those from eastern and southern Europe, Africa and Asia). (p. 8)

If there is neither innerness nor authenticity of any self or soul, and if existence, as Sartre indicated, is nothing except an accident or a chance, how can an innerness make sense? There will be no pristine self that can be achieved, as there will be no genuine innerness through which one can repose in peace.

Thus, self, soul, spirit, consciousness, innerness, inwardness, and choice are only the by-product of societal construction with a cumulative priming that can generate an illusion of sensibility; otherwise, they have no place in a robotic, mechanical world.

The significance of the abovementioned distinction may delineate how an evolutionary perspective on human nature and its ensuing biological and reductionist viewpoints can, if at all, lead to a perfunctory sense of peace. To implement this superficial sense of peace, one may apply sundry interventions from a behavioral, cognitive, or psychoanalytical perspective to only end up at a barren land of a pseudo form of peace. Both Freudian and Lacanian psychoanalysis have already pointed out the impossibility of attaining a real interpersonal and intrapersonal peace.

Not surprisingly enough, thinking, the mind, mindsets, and dysfunctional thinking have been prioritized in human scholarship in the pervasive Western models of human tranquility. The emphasis has been placed on thoughts and thinking.

CHAPTER 3

Psychology of Peace in the Outer World

Some parts of the psychological literature on peace in the mainstream Western perspective approach peace in an oppositional taxonomy with war. Accordingly, the essence of their findings focuses on ways to prevent war, manage conflict constructively, negotiate effectively, expand knowledge about parties involved in conflicts, increase the spirit of cooperation and collaboration among opposing parties, enhance the level of trust and understanding, revisit the perception of the enemy, and so forth (e.g., see Holt & Silverstein, 1989; Kelman, 1965).

Christie et al. (2008, pp. 543–544) present an elaborate record of peacekeeping, peacemaking, and peace-building strategies and make a distinction between negative and positive peace, indicating,

> [W]e focus not only on negative peace, by which we mean efforts to reduce violent episodes, but also positive peace (Galtung, 1985; Wagner, 1988), which refers to the promotion of social arrangements that reduce social, racial, gender, economic, and ecological injustices as barriers to peace. Thus, a comprehensive peace would not only eliminate overt forms of violence (negative peace) but also create a more equitable social order that meets the basic needs and rights of all people (positive peace). The pursuit of both negative and positive peace is articulated in the United Nations Educational, Scientific and Cultural Organization's (UNESCO's) definition of peace:
>
> "There can be no genuine peace when the most elementary human rights are violated, or while situations of injustice continue to exist; conversely, human rights for all cannot take root and achieve full growth while latent or open conflicts are rife. . . .
>
> Peace is incompatible with malnutrition, extreme poverty and the refusal of the rights of peoples to self-determination. Disregard for the rights of individuals and peoples, the persistence of inequitable international economic structures, interference in the internal affairs of other states, foreign occupation and apartheid are always real or potential sources of armed conflict and international crisis. The only lasting peace is a just peace based on respect for human rights" (UNESCO, 1983, pp. 259, 26).

24

By virtue of their analysis on the interpersonal, structural, cultural, and social components of conflicts, war, and peace, Christie et al. (2008) argue that

> Among the more challenging projects for peace psychology in the 21st century is to understand the conditions under which active nonviolence (negative peace) can produce socially just ends (positive peace) (Mayton, 2001, in press; Montiel, 2006). Clearly, regardless of the size of the unit of analysis (interpersonal, intergroup, or international), or setting (family, community, etc.), sustainable peace requires multilevel interventions that integrate negative and positive peace processes.

Similar works have concentrated on the exploration of peace and its oppositional counterparts – namely, war, conflict, and violence – and have proposed macro and micro interventions to remove the ferocity of violence and war and change the destructive conflicts into constructive dialogues.

Some studies have discussed the role of perception and misperception in causing conflicts and wars. Findings on the psychological implications of perception and misperception demonstrate that supposing one's assumptions are also assumed by the other party may lead to widening gaps, tension, conflicts, and wars. Similarly, in spousal life, you might presume that your partner is aware of your assumptions, but in fact he or she is unaware of them. The lack of accessibility to the other party's assumptions has contributed to the eruption of wars and conflicts.

The First World War has been historically and psychologically examined in this regard, and it is interesting to know that none of the leaders of the time were planning to wage a war. Among the most salient variables that impact the inception of war is the role of each country's perceptions. Your preparation and mobilization of forces to protect yourself at a time of threat may appear to the other party as your willingness and readiness to stage a war. The security dilemma seems to be one of the main causes of generating a perception, albeit wrong on one side, that the party is getting ready to launch a war. When a state takes precautionary measures or attempts to increase its own security, it may be purporting the opposite: decreasing the security of its neighbors.

In addition to the security dilemma, scholars have discussed the role of deterrence in explaining the onset or avoidance of conflicts. Deterrence has been described mainly as measures and attempts in the form of threats to impede the process of the opposing party's actions. Again, one may notice the significance of perception in contributing to the emergence of deterrence: both sides need to believe in the seriousness and effectiveness of the threat from the other party; otherwise, deterrence would not function correctly. The volumes of threats exchanged between the United States and the former Soviet Union during the Cold War era may exemplify one case of deterrence. As such, deterrence has been used psychologically to maintain peace between conflicting parties.

In discussing the psychological aspect of deterrence, Johnson, Mueller, and Taft (2002, p. 12) indicate that

> Deterrence, like all coercion, occurs in the mind of the adversary. Reality matters in deterrence only insofar as it affects the perceptions of those who will choose whether or not to be deterred. ... [Thus] assessments of the adversary's capabilities are of only limited predictive values unless accompanied by sound understanding of what the enemy values, how it perceives the conflict, how it makes decisions – to name but a few of the critical variables.

The psychological components of peace and war can be further studied through probing the perceptions of policy makers and decision makers in security contexts. This may elucidate the difference between objective reality and the subjective reality of the decision makers. A nation's objective reality in terms of number of weapons and military capability may not necessarily correspond to the decision makers' subjective reality.

The interplay of other psychological factors, such as stress level as a precipitating factor of conflicts, has been the subject of other studies. Some scholars have presented "democratic peace" arguments and have indicated that democracies are more favorable abodes for celebrating the reality of peace since they nurture the concept of accountability. The argument goes on to say that when there is no accountability, there is higher risk for atrocities, war, and conflicts. So the relationship between accountability and peace has been examined as another psychological variable.

Other scholarly works have focused on opposing views on war and peace with a reference to strategic history. These works have underscored the role of history in understanding current events. Strategic history refers to the history of the influence and use of force. One view has claimed that the world is moving toward peace and the absence of war, whereas the other one contends that the world will be ultimately embedded in the past strategic history, with war and conflicts all over the place (see Gray, 2007).

Gray (2007) explores the concept of war and peace in different eras and, while analyzing the historical, political, social, and economic conditions, argues that global peace cannot be established through institutional engineering. Peace requires shared understanding of cultural values and expanding a shared understanding of historical experiences. In doing so,

Gray (2007, p. 277) cites Michael Howard, who explains "why world peace cannot be constructed by the invention, or reform, of institutions":

> The establishment of a global peaceful order thus depends on the creation of a world community sharing the characteristics that make possible domestic order, and this will require the widest possible diffusion of those characteristics by the societies that already possess them. World order cannot be created simply by building international institutions and organizations that do not arise naturally out of the cultural disposition and historical experience of their members. Their creation and operation require at the very least the existence of a transnational elite that not only shares the same cultural norms but can render those norms acceptable within their own societies and can where necessary persuade their colleagues to agree to the modifications necessary to make them acceptable. (Howard, 2001, p. 105)

CHAPTER 4

Langerian Mindfulness and Peace

In addition to numerous perspectives on peace and its conditions, I present mindfulness in an independent chapter to demonstrate how mindfulness, especially Langerian mindfulness, may play a significant role in implementing peace. Before delineating how this may occur, I need to discuss the preliminary points that can provide a précis on mindfulness, its definition, different types of mindfulness, and their implications.

The Western world has witnessed two major types of mindfulness, one of which goes to meditation-based mindfulness and is associated with Jon Kabat-Zinn. This type of mindfulness, which has its roots in Buddhism, argues that meditation is the key for peace and tranquility. This perspective indicates that our desires, our wants, our yearnings, and our attachments may occupy our minds so much so that we experience a fullness and busyness in our heads. This takes away the preciousness of silence and emptiness and brings us to a world of subjective engagements, ruminations, and distractions. The more we are subjected to the tyranny of such preoccupations, the less we experience calmness, tranquility, and peace.

Kabat-Zinn (2005) emphasizes meditation practices in developing a different stance in the world, a radical shift in perspective, and "orthogonal rotation in consciousness."

In meditation-based mindfulness, meditation is introduced as the key to bringing the world of attachments and engagements into a world of presence and focus).

Studies and experiments that have operated in the heart of meditation-based mindfulness have demonstrated that meditation practices and mindful breathing meditation can help people overcome their depression, manage their stress, decrease their emotional reactivity, manage their anger, reduce their negative affectivity, and remove their tension and unrest.

Other experimental studies and interventions inspired by meditation-based mindfulness have concentrated on bringing calmness and peace by helping individuals overcome and cope with alcohol dependence, chronic pain with opiate dependence, and stress-related sleep disturbance (see Brewer et al., 2010; Garland, 2013).

Whereas the Western behavioral therapeutic perspectives have prescribed interventions including distraction, exposure, cognitive reappraisal, restructuring, controlling, and thought stopping to help people defeat their negative thoughts and their negative affects and come to peace, meditation-based mindfulness has proposed a radically different view on bringing peace to the sorrow-stricken mind or those afflicted with rumination and negativity: change how you relate to your thoughts and your mental events (e.g., see Baer, 2007; Teasdale, 1999). This different mode of relatedness is sometimes called metacognitive awareness, reperceiving, and decentering.

Meditation-based mindfulness considers meditation practice along with an observational attitude as the keys to peace and well-being. Observation espouses an empowerment to look at the inner experience without any judgments; a reactive mind removes the possibility of calmness, as it induces a sudden and reactive response. Learning meditation practices and skills of observation have helped people experience tranquility and equanimity in the face of stressful situations, challenges, and encumbrances (e.g., see Dobkin, 2008).

In line with the emergence and promotion of meditation-based mindfulness in the Western world, Herbert Benson and Richard Davidson expanded the applications and implications of the Eastern type of mindfulness in medicine and neuroscience, respectively. They underlined the monism in the mind–body relationship and demonstrated how happiness and peace can be acquired as skills. This emphasis on the interconnectedness of the mind–body relationship gave rise to numerous experimental, clinical, and medical studies that highlight the significance of learning about and training in meditation in creating a world of happiness and calmness. Whereas Benson demonstrated and argued that meditation practices can remove stress and bring calmness through developing a relaxation response (Benson, Beary, & Carol, 1974), other researchers proposed that mindfulness practices would give rise to tranquility and peace not by generating a relaxation response but by espousing mechanisms that ultimately lead to changes, rectification, and modifications of emotional and cognitive coping processes (e.g., see Ditto, Eclache, & Goldman, 2006).

When it comes to healing and psychotherapy, mindfulness has demonstrated its rigor in bringing tranquility back to patients and clients. The psychotherapeutic models operating in the realm of mindfulness include mindfulness-based stress reduction (MBSR; Kabat-Zinn, 1990), mindful cognitive modalities, mindfulness-based cognitive therapy (MBCT; Segal, Williams, & Teasdale, 2002), acceptance and commitment therapy (ACT), dialectical behavioral therapy (DBT; Dimidjian & Linehan, 2003; Linehan, 1993), and tools from other mind–body healing therapies.

The Buddhist version of mindfulness considers carving, attachment, and suffering as the main factors contributing to the dissipation of peace. When one is drastically attached to anything, becomes so preoccupied with the thought of losing anything or anyone, and suffers and experiences pain as a result of the loss or thinking about the loss, one becomes devoid of peace. To achieve peace, one needs to accept reality as it is; meditative practices teach people how to live nonjudgmentally and in the moment, without getting stuck in the meanders of thoughts, emotions, and subjective experiences. The point is to free the mind from its occupiers that impersonate the role of authenticity and to dissolve the pretentiousness of the mind's wanderings and their masks in being real.

In describing the peace-oriented moment coming out of meditation-based mindfulness and being awakened from the sleepiness of afflicted minds embroiled in tension and unrest, Hanh (1976) indicates that

> [t]he sadness or anxiety, hatred, or passion, under the gaze of our concentration and meditation, reveals its own nature. That revelation leads naturally to healing and emancipation. The sadness, or whatever, having been the cause of pain, can be used as a means of liberation from torment and suffering. We call this using a thorn to remove a thorn. We should treat our anxiety, our pain, our hatred and passion gently, respectfully, not resisting it, but living with it, making peace with it, penetrating into its nature by the meditation on interdependence.

On the power of letting go in mindfulness practices and achieving peace, Ajahn Chah says, "If you let go a little, you will have a little peace. If you let go a lot, you will have a lot of peace. If you let go completely, you will have complete peace" (Chah, Kornfield, & Breiter, 2004, as cited in Teasdale & Chaskalson, 2011).

Along with meditation-based mindfulness and its ramifications in bringing calmness, happiness, and serenity, Langerian mindfulness opens up a new version of understanding mindfulness by arguing and demonstrating that although meditation can give rise to mindfulness, one can experience mindfulness without meditation (see Langer, 1989, 2000, 2005, 2009).

Langer's empirical studies and experiments over the past 40 years offer a new view on mindfulness and its implications. Langerian mindfulness argues that our mindlessness in the world has given rise to a lack of peace and has hampered the process of living in peace. She argues that entrapment in our mindlessly created world has not allowed us to revisit the our maintained perspectives – at the cost of our wellness and well-being.

In her preface, Langer (2016) uses the analogy of bullying and says,

> Why does the bully bully? Can we see things from his perspective? Successfully pushing someone around can make us feel strong. Thus it seems mindless to me to try to put a stop to the abuse by telling bullies any version of "It's not nice to pick on the weak" since doing so makes them feel big. A mindful alternative is to teach children that only weak people bully. If they knew they'd been seen as weak, there would be little reason to bully. Changing people's behavior works better when we look at their actions from their perspective. (p. xviii)

Langer argues that the key to mindfulness begins with an intentional attempt to notice novelty. She proposes that once we look for the newness and fresh complexions of what we experience, we will experience a phenomenological sense of connectedness to the moment.

Our sense of living changes as we plan to sharpen our focus on exploring novelty as we relate to everything around us. Mindfulness, therefore, espouses an enlivening impact where one experiences exhilaration, vivacity, and livelihood. To Langer, this sense of revitalization is the panacea for peace and tranquility.

Langer explicates the role of mindfulness in bringing vitality through discussing its opposite, namely, mindlessness. Mindlessness describes a passive, automatic, and non-proactive state of mind where one is merely reacting and responding through previously learned processes. When mindless, people lose their grasp of the here and now and become circumscribed and stuck in the previous categories, experiences, emotions, thoughts, and events.

Mindlessness deprives people of accessing the newness of the moment as it filters, limits, and constricts the immediate now. In order to be disconnected from the moment, the repertoires of the past – in the forms of thoughts, emotions, memories, recollections, concepts, categorizations, classifications, taxonomy, ideas, feelings, and behaviors – seize the scope of attention so much so that they minimize the possibility of relating to the present moment. The tyranny of the past overdetermines the present moment, and thus the here and now is strongly taken by the sovereignty of the preestablished mentality and mindset.

Right at the early stages of their life, people can learn to make a distinction between themselves and everything. So they can easily distinguish between themselves as an independent entity and others and objects.

This distinction, however, is not easily made in understanding the difference between the mind and the owner of the mind. Thus, it may be hard for people to detach themselves from their mind; they tend to identify themselves with their mind. When the mind is overblown with past-stricken belongings, whether affect or cognition, it can easily impose its occupation against the present moment. The imposition does not allow the person to live in the moment and experience the now as it unfolds itself in the present time.

Langer argues that repetition and exposure to the flux of the past, whether in the form of learning and teaching or habits and styles of life, would bring mindlessness to life. A mindless way of living is characterized in an automatic, recursive, and repetitive manner where the person tends to be more reactive instead of proactive. Reactivity displays itself more in the form of habituated ways of dealing with the demands of daily life and responding to events, people, and concepts in preplanned ways.

Emotional and cognitive reactivity causes routinized styles of life to take control of decision making. Their impact is deeply traceable in interpersonal and intrapersonal relationships. The reactive way of living, to Langer, is mostly associated with affliction, passivity, tension, emotional entanglement, and paralysis of creativity. Langer considers acting from a single perspective, exposure, cultivation, and repetition, as well as an indulgence in outcome-oriented actions, as the main contributors to mindlessness.

Mindlessness espouses a passive state of mind where windows of looking at new possibilities and searches for novelty are shut down. Mindlessness operates in a dogmatic and inflexible manner whereby one's mindset is marked by stubbornness rather than openness.

Langer (1997) calls for revisiting the positions of certainty and indicates that

> [i]n a mindful state, we implicitly recognize that no one perspective optimally explains a situation. Therefore, we do not seek to select the one response that corresponds to the situation, but we recognize that there is more than one perspective on the information given and we choose from among these. (p. 108)

Langerian mindfulness argues that mindlessness prescribes an adherence to rule-governed behavior where the behavior is automatically subsumed under learned categories that present themselves as unquestionable, legitimate, and sensible.

Langer expands the exploration of mindfulness and examines how scientific postulations may fall into the traps of mindlessness:

Science, which prides itself on its objectivity, usually hides its choices from us even as it reports its findings. Many design choices that go into even our most rigorous scientific studies affect their outcomes. Greater awareness of these choices would make the findings less absolute and more useful to us. In fact, scientific research is reported in journals as probability statements, although textbooks and popular magazines often report the same results as absolute facts. This change is done to make the science easier for the nonscientists to understand. But what it does, instead, is deceive us by promoting an illusion of stability. That illusion is fostered by taking people out of the equation – what choices the researcher made in setting up the experiment, on whom it was tested, and under what circumstances. (Langer 2005, p. 106)

When patterns of automaticity reign their power and control, they proscribe any alternative ways of looking at things. In describing this mechanism, Langer indicates that sensitivity toward contexts can serve as a great avenue to change mindlessness into mindfulness. Patterns of repetition bring the illusion of sensibility and imply that their being recursive would be tied to their legitimacy and righteousness. When the mindset is replete with a plethora of repetitive patterns of thoughts, emotions, behaviors, concepts, labels, and words, this stability of thinking might give rise to the stability of the outside world.

An indulgence in and attachment to recursive subjectivity may dissolve the possibility of disengaging oneself from the realm of fixed assumptions. In delineating the hazards of such impacts, Langer (2009) posits that

[w]hen we learn mindlessly we look at experience and impose a contingent relationship between two things – what we or someone else did and what we think happened as a result. We interpret that experience from a single perspective oblivious to the other ways it can be seen. Mindful learning looks at experience and understands that it can be seen in countless ways, that new information is always available, and that more than one perspective is both possible and extremely valuable. It is an approach that leads us to be careful about what we "know" to be true and how we learn it. At the level of the particular experience, each event is unique. Why do we think we can learn from experience? That is, if events don't necessarily repeat themselves, what can one event teach us about a future event? (pp. 29–30)

When mindless, people go by routinized behaviors, habits, impulses, and emotional reactivity. This puts them in a position of inattention toward the present experience; they are more affected by their unconscious world. Their reactivity fosters the tendency to equate external events with reactive, instantaneous, and unconscious responses. So when an external event occurs, reactive responses in the form of automatic, unconscious reactions might be induced, and the appearance and manifestation of reactive responses may not be considered separable from the event.

Anxiety, tension, helplessness, desperation, and powerlessness are often the result of an incarceration in the automatic state of mind or mindlessness. Mindlessness espouses disempowerment, depression, and addiction.

Langer's experiments demonstrated that an increase of mindfulness and its consequential appreciation of multiple perspectives and viewpoints would reduce bias and judgmental attitudes (see Langer, Bashner, & Chanowitz, 1985). Langer proposes that welcoming new information and new categories can lead to mindfulness. When mindless, people remain and operate in the same old outlook that they have been exposed to, have subscribed to, or have lived through out of habituation. This enmeshment in the old categories and old conceptualizations would impose a certain bias toward not noticing new things: when you know that you know, you are not going to pay any attention to any new thing that you don't know.

Enmeshment in preexisting categories and labels would paralyze one's power to pay attention to any new thing. With one's attention frozen and imprisoned in a single perspective, one may end up adamantly refusing to welcome the possibility of a new sensibility. The adamancy of emphasizing one perspective would question the legitimacy of alternative perspectives and heighten the privilege and supremacy of one's own or one's group's perspective. Peace requires the celebration of the meaningfulness of others' beings and sensibility: their entity, their identity, and their independence.

When mindlessness reigns, openness toward new information is blocked. Understanding interpersonal, intercultural, and international relationships is replaced by a cyclic repetition of preexisting biases, judgments, and attitudes without a genuine search into the context of what the relationship is all about.

The lack of openness toward new information lessens the possibility of being receptive in dialogical interactions. When receptiveness goes away and monologism takes control of the relationship, gaps will be expanded and there will be little room to create values. Trust disappears and arrogance appears.

Mindlessness is embedded within automatic thinking and reactive responses. Negative emotions including anger, hatred, bellicosity, animosity, hostility, and bitterness induce automatic thinking that leads to mindlessness in practice. Langer's studies and experiments demonstrate that mindfulness can be linked to uncertainty and the position of not knowing.

Langer (2005, p. xvii) suggests that "when we live our lives mindlessly, we don't see, hear, taste, or experience much of what might turn lives verging on boredom into lives that are rich and exciting."

When stressed out, people may often lose their power of celebrating uncertainty and succumb to their preexisting mindsets. This may cause an inability to look at alternative ways of dealing with the situation, thus ending up in reactive, automatic reactions that are ultimately mindless. Such mindlessness is aligned with impulsive, reactive, thoughtless, and automatic responses.

In mindless behavior, there is no room for pause, revision, reframing, stopping, control, metacognition, and meta-attention. Furthermore, mindless behavior is devoid of appreciation of possibilities except for the one mindlessly derived possibility. This narrow-minded interpretation of possibility would force the actor to see himself or herself bound by a reactive response where choices are limited and limiting. If negative feelings operate in the background, the reaction would be stronger and more intense. The intensity and severity of negative feelings and emotions contribute to the emergence of an avoidance or aversion tendency, which largely serves as a preliminary element of psychological tension and turbulence. In contrast, Langerian mindfulness broadens the scope of possibility and attention to variability, thus expanding the realm of decision making in the midst of challenges and tensions.

Mindlessness brings forth the illusion that resources are limited, options are constricted, choices are minimized, and power is paralyzed. Mindlessness is associated with anxiety, fear, and powerlessness. Fear induces reactive responses, and anxiety awakens the top-down processing where the mind loses its communication with the immediate experience.

Langer's experiments demonstrated that underneath psychological tensions and conflicts, there lies the governance of mindlessness that stops people from welcoming new information, being sensitive toward context, and celebrating the possibility of multiple perspectives.

Langerian mindfulness highlights a state of mind that is connected to the moment while openly, curiously, caringly, and flexibly exploring multiple possibilities. Presence is of vital importance in Langerian mindfulness. Presence incorporates a mental, cognitive, emotional, behavioral, and fully fledged ontological and existential readiness to focus on the here and now. Langerian mindfulness proposes a foundational, radical transformation of consciousness (see Fatemi, 2014, 2016, 2018).

Authenticity and peace walk together in Langerian mindfulness. When one is disguised in pretentious and ostentatious complexions of life, one distances oneself from one's own genuine being. The more the distance between genuineness and bogusness grows, the more one falls into the experience of uneasiness and tensions.

When mindlessness reigns, absentia follows: lively connectedness to the present moment fades as the subjective maximization of the past or the future impedes the process of experiencing the present. Mindfulness blooms in presence and through presence. Presence entails wholeness and oneness: the subjective experience and the objective experience integrate with one another, and the dichotomy of the subject–object relationship ceases to operate.

Mindfulness enlivens the genius of harmony and trust. Harmony and wholeness activate one's available potentials to bloom and operate in a confident manner. When harmony and authenticity operate together, one can increase one's abilities to tranquilize one's mind, to calm one's thoughts, and to bring peace into one's awareness. Monitoring, managing, and regulating one's feelings and emotions take place in view of the heightened sense of awareness and increased ability to manage attention.

Attention may be described as the centerpiece of either tension and unrest or peace and calmness. When one's attention is aimlessly coiling around invasive thoughts and disruptive feelings and imaginations, one is often engulfed in rumination that fosters anxiety and depression.

Mindfulness teaches one to skillfully work on the quality of the mind and enhance one's power of observing thoughts, feelings, and emotions as running mental events. Understanding the transient nature of thoughts, feelings, and emotions would help one to make a discernment of the temporality of mental events; however, they are held in our minds as stable and fixed.

Questioning the unchangeability of thoughts, feelings, and emotions would usher in the possibility of detaching them from our mind. In mindlessness, we become so attached and linked to our mental events that we identify them with ourselves. This identification makes it hard for us to see that we are different from what is in our mind. The intensification of this hardship imposes the conclusion that what we feel and say to ourselves may necessarily correspond to what is out there in the real, objective world. Hypothetically speaking, then, if your mind is filled with fear and anxiety, it might follow that there should be something terrible and petrifying out there. This lack of distinction would exacerbate the situation and force one to respond to events and people based on some preexisting repertoires of mindsets, thus coming up with reactive and automatic responses. But peace does not linger in the havoc of automaticity. Peace needs to be earned in light of awareness and management of attention.

Langer (2005, p. 27) discusses the role of choices for the self and suggests that "that is the essence of a personal renaissance, to learn to act and engage with ourselves mindfully, creatively, actively, and happily." Langerian mindfulness discusses the relationship between mindfulness and creativity as the centerpiece of wellness and peace. This might resonate with Winnicott's discussion of spontaneity, where he argues that creativity and health walk together.

Mindfulness in Langerian focus also delineates the significance of seeking a flow of information from multiple perspectives. War, conflicts, skirmishes, unrest, turmoil, and turbulence can often escalate when misunderstanding, lack of understanding, indifference toward understanding, and avoiding a willingness to understand take place. Mindfulness, especially from an intercultural perspective, requires a serious attempt to reach the other party or parties involved to ensure that their message is understood and taken seriously.

This understanding, itself, needs to be mindfully shaped. For instance, creating the types of message, the way to address the audience, how to frame the intended points, how to use the words, and how to approach the audience are substantially different in high-context cultures versus low-context cultures. In low-context cultures, including Scandinavian countries, the preference goes to straightforward messages with clear-cut, lucid, and direct content. So if you happen to be thirsty there, you need to spell it out clearly, call a spade a spade, and enunciate that you need a glass of water.

On the contrary, in high-context cultures, nonverbal cues and communication, as well as the surrounding contexts, play a significant role in the meaning-making process of the message. You may hear someone saying that two-thirds of the body is composed of water, or he or she might present the differences between climatic conditions of deserts and oceans along with the ecological impacts of rain in several layers to get closer to expressing that he or she is asking for a glass of water. Similarly, when asking someone in Japan whether you can park your car in a spot, it is not just what he or she says that demonstrates the yes or no response in your situation, but it is also how he or she says it, the tone used, and so forth that clarify the response behind his or her intention.

When speaking of mindfulness and understanding, one needs to be aware of the types of understanding, the context of understanding, the layers of understanding, and the surrounding facets of understanding. An increased sense of mindful understanding may allow one to revisit the labels, preexisting mental concepts, prejudgmental propositions, unquestionably accepted analyses, taken-for-granted responses, and automatic reactions.

Langer and Abelson's (1974) study, "A Patient by Any Other Name," may exemplify how the legitimacy of one perspective known as expert can take control over other perspectives. According to the study, clinicians representing behavioral and analytic schools of thought (i.e., two groups of "experts") viewed a single videotaped interview between a man who had recently applied for a new job and one of the authors. One half of each group was told that the interviewee was a "job applicant," whereas the remaining half was told that he was a "patient." At the end of the videotape, all clinicians were asked to complete a questionnaire evaluating the interviewee. The interviewee was described as fairly well adjusted by the behavioral therapists regardless of the label supplied. This was not the case, however, for the more traditional therapists. When the interviewee was labeled "patient," he was described as significantly more disturbed than he was when he was labeled "job applicant."

In elucidating the impacts and functions of labels in bringing mindlessness, Langer (2009) explains that

> [l]abels lead us to go on hypothesis-confirming data searches. That is, we look for evidence to support the label. Since most information is ambiguous, the result is "seek and ye shall find." The label "patient" leads us to examine behavior and life circumstances through a problem-finding lens. The label "patient" also leads us and doctors to search for illness related symptoms. In both cases, behavior and sensations from the norm are interpreted as unhealthy. Moreover, independent cues of health may be totally ignored. (p. 135)

Lack of mindful understanding, passive reliance on transposed and transferred assumptions, learning in the clinical world dealing with the cure for tension, and concern for wellness and health have also widened the gaps between the reality of clients' and patients' lives and the given instructions.

In exposing the failure of these labels and mindlessly taken approaches, Linley and Joseph (2004) argue that

> these assumptions are typically implicit, and therefore are often uncritically accepted by practitioners trained in a particular model and a particular way of knowing. It is precisely because these fundamental assumptions are implicit that they are so often taken for granted and unchallenged, assuming the position of the status quo. (p. 714)

Langer (2009) points out the perils of mindless underendowing in prescribing instructions before doing mindful diagnosis and says that

> [w]e would be aware that medical facts are not handed down from the heavens, but in fact are determined by people under changing, different conditions. I don't think I can say often enough that medical decisions rest on uncertainty – if there were no uncertainty, there would be no decision to be made. To reveal at least some of this uncertainty would mean that while our doctors may be knowing and caring, they cannot be all-knowing. They are subject to the same biases and value-based judgments as the rest of us. But doctors often feel they have to hide their uncertainty. (p. 136)

In revisiting the absolute oriented statements versus conditional statements in the psychological research, Teo (2018) argues that

> [e]mpirical psychologists present theoretical interpretations of empirical statements as facts or knowledge to the scientific community or the public. Yet, the fact that statements about race differences, for instance, contain speculations and theoretical interpretations is not conveyed to the public. An empirical result of difference in a psychological characteristic depends on the questions asked, the instruments and methods used, and the assumptions made, but it also depends on the meaning that is given to differences, and on whether they are attributed to an essence, nature, or culture. The discussion of the empirical result is not determined by data (but based on data) and requires a hermeneutic process that is undervalued and not taught in the discipline and profession of psychology. (p. 221)

Langer argues that mindlessness gives rise to tension and unrest and blocks the possibility of exploring liberating alternatives. Langer's (2009, p. 18) psychology of possibility targets the mindsets and their stability as the commencement of exploring the possibility of change as she iterates that "we imagine the stability of our mindsets to be the stability of the underlying phenomena and so we don't think to consider the alternatives."

Langer's focus on possibility goes beyond the epistemological possibility and highlights the significance of ontological possibility. The roadblocks, Langer argues, to understanding ontological possibility happen in the realm of epistemology, where the commitment to specific epistemological propositions hampers exploring the avenues of new possibilities.

Langer focuses on the paralyzing power of cognitions when they tend to stabilize their certitude in view of their frequency, repetition, cultivation, and socialization. Langer indicates how possibility can be limited and limiting when one is forcibly circumscribed in the prescriptive and proscriptive modes of possibility. The leap from the limiting sense of possibility to the liberating sense of possibility, according to Langer, begins with questioning the province of possibility, namely, the mindsets that describe the realm of possibility. Through her experiments, Langer questions the borders of possibility and revisits the quantifiers of propositional possibilities in which certain quantifiers are known to apply for acknowledging certain possibilities.

Mindlessness, according to Langer, paralyzes our power of choices and imposes passive and automatic behaviors. Through our mindlessness, we depreciate the value of our being a human as we lose our sense of control over what we do and how we do it. Langer examines the interplay of tension, anxiety, and mindlessness and uses the term *authentic selves* to consider mindlessness as the roadblock that prevents us from experiencing the genuine and authentic self. When authenticity is dissipated, she argues, calmness fades away. Mindful understanding of the perspective of others requires an understanding of both their rational and experiential mind. The rational mind consists of the analytical mind where information processing takes place through syllogism, inferential thinking, evidence, reasoning, and conscious efforts, whereas the experiential mind operates in the scope of one's experiences and one's own unconscious world (see Pacini & Epstein, 1999).

A superficial understanding may only proceed with an exploration of someone's linear and analytical mind. On the rational level, one may be convinced to undertake or avoid a behavior, but when it comes to the experiential level, one may find it hard to see the implications in practice. We may try to see someone's world by stepping into his or her logical and analytical mind without approaching his or her experiential world.

In conflicts resolution, in therapy, and in mediation, we may apprehend what someone's mind is saying on the rational level. However, we may fail to reach him or her in terms of his or her experiential sphere.

Langerian mindfulness proposes that understanding multiple perspectives would bring a new horizon of awareness where creating values could occur. Creating values would entail a focus on common grounds, establishing trust and empathy, and building bridges by finding areas of mutual interest.

Understanding mindfully also involves an interplay of communicative action in the world of the actor. In other words, if the world of the perceiver is blocked by his or her preexisting judgments and assumptions, the world of the other is mindlessly distorted. Understanding mindfully thus requires an act of self-reflection and detachment, which includes putting away one's presuppositions and going beyond one's collections of knowing.

Sensitivity to context, in Langerian mindfulness, refers to this openness and flexibility in reaching the world of the other. Langer argues that our mindlessness can be deeply rooted in our long-lived mindsets, which can impose restrictive measures against our success, our novelty, and our well-being.

Langer (2009) indicates,

> In more than thirty years of research, I've discovered a very important truth about human psychology: certainty is a cruel mindset. It hardens our minds against possibility and closes them to the world we actually live in. When all is certain, there are no choices for us. If there is no doubt, there is no choice. When we are certain, we are blind to the uncertainties of the world whether we recognize it or not. It is uncertainty that we need to embrace, particularly about our health. If we do so, the payoff is that we create choices and the opportunity to exercise control over our lives. (pp. 24–25)

Kierkegaard (1992) explicates the importance of mindfulness toward the actor's perspective in a wide variety of contexts. He demonstrates how superiority within the observer's perspective can be detrimental in communicating the truth and suggests,

> Take the case of a man who is passionately angry, and let us assume that he is really in the wrong. Unless you can begin with him by making it seem that it were he who had to instruct you, and unless you can do it in such a way that the angry man, who was too impatient to listen to a word of yours, is glad to discover in you a complacent and attentive listener – if you cannot do that, you cannot help him at all. Or take the case of a lover who has been unhappy in love, and suppose that the way he yields to his passions is really unreasonable, impious, unchristian. In case you cannot begin with him in such a way that he finds genuine relief in talking to you about his suffering and is able to enrich his mind with the poetical interpretations you suggest for it, notwithstanding you have no share in this passion and want it to free him from it – if you cannot do that, then you cannot help him at all; he shuts himself away from you, he retires within himself . . . and then you just talk at him. (p. 45)

In line with the presentation of a rigorous analysis on the inner conflicts, internal tension, and intrapersonal and interpersonal pandemonium, Schneider (2018) focuses on fear and anxiety and their operative mode in giving rise to the polarized mind, where one experiences "the fixation on a single point of view to the utter exclusion of competing points of view." The fixation gives rise to a dogmatic approach when one turns out to be adamant and recalcitrant toward accepting anything other than one's own view.

Schneider argues that the experience of trauma, abuse, molestation, and other physical and psychological pain may often lead to the production of anxiety and fear. The excruciatingly painful experiences may belong to both one's personal and collective past, and thus we may witness the operation of the polarized mind at both the individual and societal levels.

In both layers of personhood and societal manifestations, the polarized mind may also reflect a reaction against the feeling of incompetence, insignificance, worthlessness, shame, groundlessness, and negligence. The reaction may unfold itself in a heightened sense of a grandiose, presumptuous, overbearing attitude and self-centeredness with an idiosyncratic sense of dogmatism where one is deeply indulged in one's righteousness and leaves one's certainty unquestionable. Correspondingly, the fear- and anxiety-driven mind might turn out to be violent and demonstrate extremism, racism, classism, ethnocentrism, tyranny, and other societal malaise.

Schneider explores the root causes of conflicts and war across cultures and indicates that the experience of pain and trauma, abuse, and exploitation, as well as the interplay of anxiety and fear along with their ensuing feelings of incompetence, may converge and interactively produce a persistently dogmatic mindset where the legitimacy, privilege, and superiority of a monopolized perspective might emerge.

In the meantime, the polarized mind is based on the seeds of mindlessness where the reactive responses and instinctual drives and motivations intertwine with habits and repetitions (see Schneider & Fatemi, 2019).

The polarized mind's doctrine extrapolates that peace cannot be established in a climate of anxiety and fear, just as it does not grow in a land of selfishness, solipsism, despotism, extremism, and dogmatism. In order to experience peace, people need to emancipate themselves from the manacles of polarization of their mind.

Schneider's conceptualization of the polarized mind is enriched through his psychological analysis of the intrapersonal elements of conflict, fear, and anxiety. In explicating the nature of the polarized mind, Schneider (2013) says,

> Polarization, the wholesale privileging of one reality to the utter exclusion of competing realities, is one of the chief scourges of humanity. Polarization is responsible for countless deaths, degradations, and breakdowns, and its impact extends to all levels of humanity – personal, collective, psychological and spiritual. Cosmic insignificance, helplessness, and groundlessness, are at the root of the polarized mind. . . . Cosmic insignificance arises from personal and collective trauma, ignorance and fear part of which appears to be inherent to mortal life." (pp. 160–161).

In highlighting the significance of presence, Schneider (2013) indicates that

> [t]he whole-bodied awareness of the awesome conditions of life means awareness of our smallness (e.g., fragility) as well as greatness (e.g., participation) in these conditions. It also means the awareness of life's

paradoxes. . ... The acknowledgment of life's paradoxes begins with presence, which is the heightened whole-bodied awareness of the world around and within one . . ... Presence is a precursor to awe, the humility and wonder – or sense of adventure – toward living. And awe is the scaffolding for wisdom. . ... Wisdom is the guidance system for awe and leads to the fluidly centered life. This is a life that is both pliable (fluid) and contained (centered) as context and circumstance demand. (p. 161).

CHAPTER 5

Psychological Peace Finders

Discussions on how to bring peace for both interpersonal and intrapersonal realms have been influenced by psychological inquiries. This has also been associated with the implication that peace can be given and prescribed, and instructions can be offered to give rise to a peaceful world where tension goes away and calmness arrives. The conceptualization of peace as a prescriptive formula has presupposed a postulation where the knower would be able to discern the implementation of peace and would have access to the ways and workings of establishing peace. The implication has further purported that by having the right knowledge of the phenomena, applying the right method of inquiry, and ensuring the right verification method, one can encompass the right diagnosis to come up with the right prescription. The righteousness of the right techniques was considered as the panacea for dealing with the practical aspects of life, including producing peace.

Habermas has critiqued the Western approach toward understanding human problems and has suggested that technological consciousness equipped with the application of the right methods and an indulgence in instrumentalism has led to people's deprivation of reflexive and reflective thinking over their destiny and their divorce from a real contribution in fulfilling a responsible, creative role. This can obviously distort the image of peace in both the inner and the outer world.

Habermas (1975) discusses the implications of modern life at the mercy of techniques and experts and argues how knowing is forcibly contained and entrapped by the flux of techniques. In presenting his arguments, he states,

> Yet even a civilization that has been rendered scientific is not granted dispensation from practical questions: therefore a peculiar danger arises when the process of scientification transgresses the limit of reflection of a rationality confined to technological horizon. For then no attempt at all is made to attain a rational consensus on the part of citizens concerned

with the practical control of their destiny. Its place is taken by the attempt to attain technical control over history by perfecting the administration of society, an attempt that is just as impractical as it is unhistorical. (p. 255)

Correspondingly, mainstream psychology has claimed that it can define, explain, and predict peace-oriented behavior by virtue of the universally accepted linear methods of thinking. I argue that linear methods of thinking only constitute one mode of thinking, and they cannot explain the wide variety of possible modes of thinking. The presence of meanings and intentions are not taken into consideration. If the reference points that tend to understand meanings are already preoccupied within a certain domination of the signification, how could they ever help us explore the meanings? The reaction against the specific imposition of meaning within mainstream positivist psychology can be found in the works that demonstrate a challenge against the stability of meaning within one specific reference point (see Derrida, 1976; Gergen, 1990; Levy & Langer, 1994; Lotringer, 1996; Lyotard, 1984; Merryfield, 2009; Wittgenstein, 1968).

This has deep roots in the discourse of the expert in mainstream psychology and in the Western research paradigm that privileges specific voices over others by highlighting the legitimacy of a given methodology. Katz (1992) discusses how the discourse of the expert in the North American mainstream inquiry is tied to an implicit confirmation of domination and power and represents the actor or the other through the lens of the very domination. The actor's or the other's representation, she argues, is reconstructed in the context of the domineering position. Katz (1992) indicates how otherness of the other is transformed through the paradigmatic and syntagmatic prescription of the discourse of power.

Walsh-Bowers (2005) elucidates the domineering position of the researcher and articulates that

> North American psychologists' habitual adherence to a research relationship of expert investigator and ignorant "subject" had a marked impact after World War II on the rapidly expanding field of clinical psychology and ultimately on community psychology. When they adopted the "scientist-practitioner model" in 1949, clinical psychologists hoped to establish the scientific legitimacy of their profession for which identification with the hierarchical laboratory model of experimentation seemed essential. (pp. 100–101)

Demonstrating the interplay of power and politics in influencing the scientific discourse, Teo (2018) states that

[a]s widely documented (e.g., Hoffman et al., 2015), psychologists participated in the American War on Terror with enhanced interrogation techniques (i.e., torture strategies such as waterboarding). Not only did the APA not object to these practices, it was quick to abandon its principles under the Bush presidency (and beyond), ostensibly in the name of national security, and when it began rewriting the code in order to make participation in enhanced interrogation practices more easily attainable.

The preemptive obedience that the APA displayed contrasts with the American Psychiatric Association, which advised its members not to participate in enhanced interrogations, with the American Medical Association, and with the American Anthropological Association, which objected to the use of anthropologic knowledge in interrogations. Why was psychology's stance so different?

Feminist researchers have also argued that the domineering role of the researcher in psychology has led to marginalization of the subject of research and ignored the role of power, privilege, voice, equality, and subjectivity in the process of research and its implications for the subject of research (see Fine, 1992; Lather, 1991; Maher, 1999; Reinharz, 1992).

In challenging the domineering role of specific voices and highlighting the voices of the marginalized in modes of expressiveness, Fine (2002) argues that

[f]or better or worse, the more troubling question for critical feminist researchers, with respect to the presence of an absence, is not actually which methods to apply but questions about our disciplinary reliance on positivism. That is, psychology's obsession with the observable, the model-able, and the connectable has forced us into very narrow holes about what we can speak about with authority. (p. 19)

Explicating the relationship between the researcher and the subject of research within the paradigm of the expert/scientific perspective, Katz (1992) notes that

[b]uilding from feminist, postcolonial, and post structural theories the question of subject position becomes central to a new ethnography in which difference is used productively to question the multiple forms of dominance, exploitation, and oppression. (p. 504)

Langer (1997) argues that incarceration within the expert's perspective would prevent us from exploring the meanings both in core and marginal levels. The focus on signification from the expert's perspective would not allow us to revisit the reference point through which the expert's perspective is bound. Neither would it allow us to highlight or minimize the experience of the observation.

The expert's perspective within logical positivism has marginalized or ignored the personal meanings that unfold within subcultures and merely emphasize the legitimacy of the expert's perspective. The salience of the expert's role as the truth finder is associated with both cognitive and emotional impacts in that the subject of research, who is exposed to the vociferousness of the expert's voice, may not take it upon himself or herself to voice his or her presence in the meanders of the hegemony of the expert's control.

The perspective of the expert can impede the process of understanding in that it limits our understanding. In other words, understanding does not happen, as the perspective of the expert declares its reign. Instead, the expert's perspective is only an imposition of a communicative form disguised in the appearance of understanding. The perspective of the expert is one among many others, but when legitimacy is established for the single expert's perspective, other perspectives are nullified and marginalized. The view that there is an expert's perspective that needs to be legitimized is tantamount to generalizing one perspective over so many other possible perspectives.

Elaborating on the utilitarian and materialistic nature of mainstream psychology in dealing with human problems and human challenges, Teo (2018) indicates that

> [i]t is important to point out that pragmatic-utilitarian reasoning is useful in many situations of daily life (e.g., the car broke down – what should I do?). But there is also a trend in Western culture, adding a critical-historical dimension, that pragmatic-utilitarian thinking has become dominant, which is grounded in the development of political economy and its latest incarnation, neoliberalism. It is also important to point out that ethical and moral answers to the question "what should I do?" can be in contradiction. From an ethical standpoint "I" could argue that "I want to be the best father that I can be" (again, I use the "I" form as a general and not personal pronoun), who wants the best for "my" children. Thus, "I" decided, when it came to making a practical decision, to send "my" children to a private school. This decision can be ethical, but from a moral perspective, one should ask oneself about the generalizability of this decision, considering the people who cannot afford to send their children to private school, and the educational implications for other children, or for public education. From such a perspective, this decision might not be moral at all. If one adds cost–benefit analyses to the question "what should I do?" one may also add a pragmatic-utilitarian reason to the debate, such that private school is easy to afford based on "my" salary or wealth, and it gives "my" children an advantage in a competitive economy. (p. 182)

Teo (2005) demonstrates how mainstream psychology has conversely not moved in line with creating authentic peace and tranquility through its biases and manipulations, and more over adopting racists approaches. In delineating his arguments, Teo (2005) states that

> Psychology has been transformed from a philosophical into a natural scientific discipline on the background of colonialism, slavery, and exploitation. Thus, it is not surprising that important pioneers of psychology assimilated or actively contributed to scientific racism. Paul Broca (1824–1880), who is celebrated in psychology for his location of speech loss (aphasia) in an area of the brain (known as Broca's area), was one of the leaders of scientific racism. He was convinced that non-European races were inferior in terms of intelligence, vigor and beauty (see Teo 2005). It is also remarkable that Broca gave up all standards of scientific inquiry when he "handled" research on human "races." At the beginning were his conclusions, which were followed by data collection and selective reports. Criteria were changed and abandoned when the results did not fit his original conclusions (see Gould 1996). He embraced "confirming" evidence and repressed disconfirming information. The pioneer of social psychology Gustave Le Bon (1841–1931), who divided, based on psychological criteria, humans into primitive, inferior, average, and superior races, suggested vehemently that races were physiologically and psychologically distinct, that races were different species, and that all members of a race shared an immutable race soul (see Teo 2005). (pp. 154–157)

Elucidating an example that illustrates an entirely different direction against the essence of peace, Albee (1981, as cited in Nelson & Prilleltensky, 2005) highlights the 1923 statements of a Princeton psychologist, Brigham, who acts from the perspective of the observer and leaves no room for the actor. The psychologist states,

> We face the possibility of racial admixture here that is infinitely worse than that favoured by any European country today, for we are incorporating the Negro into our racial stock, while all of Europe is comparatively free from this taint. . . .. The decline of American intelligence will be more rapid . . . owing to the presence of the Negro. ()

The promotion of the knower's legitimacy and privilege in the psychological sphere has silenced the possibility of questioning the nature and dynamics of psychological power. The position of science as the decision maker and a reliable source for bringing peace and tranquility to the world of human beings and the world in general has rarely left any room for addressing the sources. In elaborating the implications of the psychological experts' assigned privilege to lead in their domineering role, Latour (2004) argues that

[o]nly in the name of science is Stanley Milgram's experiment possible, to take one of Stengers and Despret's topoi. In any other situation, the students would have punched Milgram in the face ... thus displaying a very sturdy and widely understood disobedience to authority. That students went along with Milgram's torture does not prove they harboured some built-in tendency to violence, but demonstrates only the capacity of scientists to produce artifacts no other authority can manage to obtain, because they are undetectable. The proof of this is that Milgram died not realizing that his experiment had proven nothing about average American inner tendency to obey – except that they could give the appearance of obeying white coats! Yes, artifacts can be obtained in the name of science, but this is not itself a scientific result, it is a consequence of the way science is handled (see the remarkable case of Glickman 2000). (p. 222)

The subtlety of understanding the assigned privilege of discovering the truth reveals a vital point, namely, the investigator's role in determining the levels and contents of knowing.

On the strength of an interesting analogy, Danziger (1990) indicates that

[t]he received view is based on a model of science that is reminiscent of the tale of Sleeping Beauty. The objects with which psychological science deals are all present in nature fully formed, and all the prince-investigator has to do is to find them and awaken them with the magic kiss of his research. . ... In the past the effects of a naive empiricism may have assigned an essentially passive role to investigators, as though they merely had to observe or register what went on outside them. (p. 2)

The idea of offering a prescription both for internal and external realms of human beings may need to be explored in the scientific model of knowing in mainstream psychology. The model is tied to the notion of prediction and control, and it endorses the legitimacy of the expert's perspective over that of the actor. This is the observer (i.e., the researcher) who, through using the right methods and tools, can identify not only the reality of the actor but also the needs of the actor. The actor can come to the reality of his or her problem, wants, motives, and so on through the help of the observer–researcher.

In a critique on positivist research, Code (1995) challenges the view since "knowers are detached and neutral spectators, and objects of knowledge are separate from them, inert items in knowledge-gathering processes, yielding knowledge best verified by appeals to observational data" (p. 17).

When knowers equipped with the standard language of positivist psychology are supposed to bring peace and tranquility, they may ignore the local contexts, cultural features, and specificity of situational analyses.

In a critique against the sovereignty of positivist psychology's approach, Walsh-Bowers (2005, p. 98) argues that "proponents of scientific rigor successfully imposed standards of decontextualized detachment for the investigative situation, minimizing the interpersonal context of conducting research to establish universal laws of behavior that transcended time, place, and person." Teo (2005) expands on the critique and states that

> [f]rom a critical perspective, one would have to describe an investigative practice that conceptualizes the subject matter by the way the method prescribes it, as methodologism (Teo 2005), a concept similar to the one used by Bakan (1961/1967), methodolatry (p. 158), to denote the worship of method. In a similar vein, Toulmin and Leary (1985) referred to the cult of empiricism and Danziger (1990) called it the methodological imperative. (p. 36)

The sovereignty of the positivist worldview in psychological research excluded any language and discourse that could not be apprehended through the five physical senses. One may track down the roots of positivist-driven psychology in Darwinian evolutionary theory, the privilege of the natural sciences' methodology, and their implications for formulating the universal truths (see Scruton, 2009). Psychology, in its mainstream positivist version, thus claimed to be a value-free discipline that is in search of the truth through conducting objective research with a focus on measurement. The claim purported that with the rise of the right and legitimate methodology, one can acquire the true knowledge about individuals regardless of culture, history, and contexts.

Habermas (1972) indicates that positivism monopolizes the realm of knowing and refutes the possibility of any mode of knowing except the ones that are legitimized through positivist science. In challenging positivism, Habermas (1972) indicates that "scientism means science's belief in itself: that is, the conviction that we can no longer understand science as one form of possible knowledge, but rather must identify knowledge with science" (p. 4).

With an aspiration to produce a physic like psychology that can apply the right method and can predict and control behavior, experimental psychological research contributed to the expanding assumptions that human nature can be objectively investigated. Describing the picture, Winston (2001) explicated that

> Titchener characterized Mach's view as allowing that psychology could become an exact science in the same way as physics. According to Titchener, Mach quoted Queteleton the idea that experiments "yielded

varied outcomes because of chance" but that chance is subject to law, and the "intellectual elements of our social life, the psychological processes, are no less uniform than the rest. (p. 130)

This has had significant implications for demonstrating the hidden and ulterior impediments to achieving an authentic peace in both the intrapersonal and interpersonal levels.

To exemplify this point, the researcher's voice and its legitimacy in deciding what to do have been leading factors in endorsing policies, programs, and projects with huge social implications. The proponents of IQ tests abided by social Darwinism and claimed that the ones with low intelligence were doomed to failure and had to be eradicated. The Darwinian-driven psychology considered its right to condemn those who did not possess the required intelligence (see Albee, 1981; Clark, 1965; Nelson & Prilleltensky, 2005).

Citing Laungani's objection against mainstream psychology's research and its paradigmatic leadership, Teo (2005) indicates that

> [a]ccording to Laungani, neither experimental studies not psychometric instruments nor taxonomies provide knowledge of mental life's specificity in other cultures. Laungani even goes so far as to suggest that the experiment may be a "fruitless exercise" (p. 395) in other cultures, because people may not have been socialized into the meaning of psychological-experiments. (p. 161)

The monolithic view on human beings within the domination of taken-for-granted research methodology and marginalization of research subjects and their voices has contributed to the creation of imbroglios in addressing the challenges and problems of both groups and individuals at local and international levels. In other words, this has prevented the achievability of an authentic peace.

The following quote from Sheik Muhammad Hussain Fadlallah, the spiritual leader of Lebanese Hezbollah (as cited in Ginges et al., 2011) may exemplify the gaps between the array of seemingly plausible data of the psychological observer as the expert and the reality of the actor:

> The problem with the discipline of psychology is that it attempts to study the phenomenon of martyrdom from the perspective of pragmatic vocabulary and laboratory results. They refuse to admit that certain things can be understood only through labor and pain. You can never be capable of appreciating freedom if you do not come to grips with enslavement. You can appreciate the crisis of the starved when you come to grips with the pangs of starvations. (Abu-Rabi, 1996, p. 242)

In describing and discussing how power and politics have contributed to the growth of one-sided psychological research that may not be in touch with the phenomenologically lived experiences of real people, Teo (2018) states that

> [a]nother example of pragmatic-utilitarian thinking having primacy over ethics and morality is the now widely documented financial conflict of interest issues that plague clinical psychology, psychiatry, psychotherapy, and psychoanalysis, in the context of working with the Diagnostic and Statistical Manual (DSM) (e.g., American Psychiatric Association, 2000, 2013). Cosgrove and her colleagues identified significant financial ties between the pharmaceutical industry, researchers, and panel members, who developed and advanced the manual for mental illness as well as practice guidelines (Cosgrove, Bursztajn, Krimsky, Anaya, & Walker, 2009; Cosgrove & Krimsky, 2012; Cosgrove, Krimsky, Vijayaraghavan, & Schneider, 2006; Cosgrove & Wheeler, 2013). The authors showed in their 2006 article that the majority of the 170 DSM panel members had financial links to the pharmaceutical industry, and that the relationship between money and knowledge is exacerbated in areas where drugs are considered the primary form of treatment. Despite the systematic and empirically evidenced critiques, and the well-intended improved disclosure policies, the number of financial conflicts has not declined in recent years. (p. 187)

Teo (2018) elaborates the underlying components of mainstream psychology as it unfolds itself as a science and demonstrates how, for the sake of being called a science, psychology does not openly decompose and deconstruct its taken-for-granted postulations and assumptions. He demonstrates how psychology's separation from humanities, which has been opulently helpful in the past, has imposed sundry forms of reductionism.

In line with a critique of the so-called scientific understanding of human subjectivity, Teo (2018) corroborates how psychological science has failed to fathom the multifaceted nature of human beings and has stopped in its own assumptions. This has given rise to perfunctory solutions that have touched upon a fragmented human being incarcerated in the compartmentalized technical models. Teo (2018) calls for revitalizing psychology with an inclusion of psychological humanities and an openness to going beyond the taken-for-granted scientific axioms.

Presenting a rigorous analysis of mainstream psychology's embeddedness within social, historical, cultural, economic, and political contexts, Teo (2018) provides us with an in-depth understanding of why psychological theories and psychotherapeutic interventions, albeit effective in limited layers of contexts, have been unable to assist people in our world today in creating an authentic, genuine peace in both the intrapersonal and interpersonal levels.

In discussing some of the manifest parochialism and pitfalls within mainstream psychological investigation and its worldview, Teo (2018) states that

> [b]ecause of the intrinsic relationship between psychology and contemporary society, alternative concepts and theories are required, which could still be trapped in forms of psychologization. Thus, it is crucial to assess critical psychology, which emphasizes the importance of alternative forms of agency (Holzkamp, 1983); Lacanians who question psychologists' collaborations with power (Malone, 2012; Parker, 2011; Pavón-Cuéllar, 2013); sociological psychologists (Davies, 2015; Ward, 2002) who may underestimate agency; or philosophical psychologists who look for tradition as an alternative (e.g., Smith, 2009, on alternatives to empirically supported therapies). Resistance within psychology may be futile if it does not take dialectical historical, social, (sub)cultural, and individual meanings and relationships into account (see also Papadopoulos, 2008). (pp. 230, 231)

In challenging the mainstream psychological worldview and its emphasis on the plausibility of its paradigm and the exclusion and insensibility of other paradigms, Marsella and Higginbotham (1984) indicate that

> [t]he argument that Western approaches are scientifically based while indigenous or traditional approaches are based on magic and superstition is invalid because it mistakes technology for science and because it assumes that only "rational" thinking guides Western assumptions and techniques. Further, it ignores centuries of effective healing knowledge. (p. 183)

Correspondingly, Marsella and Yamada (2007) argue that establishing interpersonal and intrapersonal wellness cannot occur without attention to socioeconomic justice, indicating the interplay of health and justice in broader context. They describe the relationship by pointing out that

> [t]here can be no mental health where there is powerlessness, because powerlessness breeds despair; there can be no mental health where there is poverty, because poverty breeds hopelessness; there can be no mental health where there is inequality, because inequality breeds anger and resentment; there can be no mental health where there is racism, because racism breeds low self-esteem and self-denigration. (p. 812)

The Western worldview on establishing inner peace has been associated with a series of challenges: It has been operating mainly from a linear, analytical, mathematical, mechanical, and reductionist model and has failed to take into consideration the interplay of complexities within human nature. It has been built on an animalistic model that has explained human behavior and the dynamics of human psychology more in terms of physiological, neurological, and bodily oriented interpretations. It has often been mindless of the contextual and situational factors and has not paid serious attention to sociopolitical, economic, and cultural factors that can affect the process of achieving peace.

The paradigmatic sovereignty of the positivist model has silenced and marginalized the alternative voices that can contribute to understanding peace beyond the mechanical model. The Western view has also been influenced by the dialectics of power and politics and has been called away from a genuine focus on exploring peace beyond political and economic interests.

CHAPTER 6

Peace and Innerness

Exploring the psychology of inner peace is ineluctably tied to an examination of the nature of innerness. If innerness is merely a by-product of neurological and physiological responses and activities, strategies to bring peace would be embedded within the same routes, namely, brain- and body-oriented channels.

On the other hand, scrutinizing the psychological aspects and nature of peace would need to ultimately address the nature of human beings. If human beings' nature is solely built upon a secular worldview, the corollary of finding remedies for a turbulent self would substantively differ from an alternative view where humanness is not summed up in the material world.

Correspondingly, if achieving peace requires the interplay of social, economic, cultural, political, and psychological factors, the conceptualization of subjectivity, agency, and empowerment would display their distinctions from a system of thought where situational components and contexts are given low priority. Furthermore, if the subject matter of an inner peace goes back to defining the characteristics of what makes a human being a human being, then a discussion on inner peace needs to address the idiosyncrasies of humanness and delve into the quiddity of the self.

It may be in line with reflecting on the nature of human beings that William James (1971) wrote,

> There are possibilities [in us] that take our breath away of another kind of happiness and power based on giving up our own will and letting something higher work for us, and these seem to show a world wider than either physics or philistine ethics can imagine. Here is a world in which all is well. (p. 266)

The Western discussion on the nature of human beings and its psychological implications has been mainly influenced by a mechanical, materialistic, and machine-oriented perspective.

Presenting a rigorous analysis on the history of psychological scholarship on humanness, Teo (2018, p. 75) examines the limitations of Western psychological approach on defining the human nature and indicates,

> Despite the fact that the psychological humanities have played a role in the self-understandings of humans, scientific psychology has thrived on explicit and implicit mechanistic ideas of human nature. Concepts are explicit when, with the development of technologies and devices, scientific psychology prepares the way to understand humans as machines from clocks, steam engines, radios, to computers (see Boden, 2006; Herzog, 1984). They are implicit in the sense that, despite a commitment to a biological model of human nature, research is exhausted methodologically in a mechanistic model. That is, certain methodologies used in psychology embody a mechanistic model (my data are not considered relevant if I walk out of an experiment that is problematic to me) and accepting a certain methodology that allows only a range of reactions implies a mechanistic theory of human nature. Such an approach may be helpful in certain situations, but does not do justice to the complexities of what it means to be human (Smith, 2007).

This nexus of ontology and methodology, or of mechanistic, atomistic, and reductionist views on what it means to be human and an experimental–analytical framework, allowed for a thriving critique of scientific psychology because of its obvious limitations to reflexive observers. Representing human subjectivity based on technological or mechanical models, and focusing on variables and on isolated aspects of human mental life, prevents an understanding of the integrated character of the mind in concrete individuals' conduct of everyday life, which always takes place in history, culture, and society.

Marsella and Higginbotham critique the Western worldview on humanness and posit that

> the argument that Western approaches are scientifically based while indigenous or traditional approaches are based on magic and superstition is invalid because it mistakes technology for science and because it assumes that only "rational" thinking guides Western assumptions and techniques. Further, it ignores centuries of effective healing knowledge. (1984, p. 183)

In presenting an alternative view on humanness and a self being distinct from the bodily oriented self, Kierkegaard tells the story of a lily "more beautifully clothed than Solomon in all his glory," who was "joyful and free of care all the day long" (1998a, 1998b). The lily, Kierkegaard narrates, is influenced by a "naughty little bird" that induces comparison by reporting on beautiful flowers in other places where the birds come up with the best songs ever. The lily begins to loathe itself and allows the bird to take it to those glorious places. Thus, in going with the bird, the lily is detached from the soil, where it belongs. Along the way, the lily perishes.

According to Kierkegaard, the lily symbolizes human beings and the naughty little bird represents the comparisons that entangle them. The soil typifies roots and connectedness. Langer presents experiments and cases that indicate how comparison-induced malaise may prevent one from exploring authentic modes of living and expressiveness.

In discussing the realm of innerness and its capacities, Kierkegaard discusses possibility as a unique, distinctly human feature that can transpire in different levels of existence and bring about different ways of living. Human beings are the only creatures, in Kierkegaard's view on possibility, who can go beyond the biologically established configuration and experience possibilities. Each realm of existence unfolds a different aspect of possibility.

The aesthete indulges in the spectrum of possibilities, playfully experiencing possibilities as he experiences the joys and pleasures of life, whether physical beauty or intellectual enjoyments. In this stage of being and possibility, the aesthete is overwhelmed by a hedonistic predisposition toward possibilities, without which his life would be devoid of any meaning. His freedom is ontologically concealed to oblivion to the effect that he solely thinks of possibilities and their infinite, unconstrained, and unlimited expansion.

In the ethical stage of possibilities, the ethical person takes responsibility and acknowledges the power of freedom and decision making. The ethical person, according to Kierkegaard, understands the limitations of possibilities as she experiences a moral way of living. This stage of possibility can be induced by either an inner or external sense of values. It can be epitomized in one's obedience to her own inner voice, in the exterior manifestations of law-abiding attitudes, or in the accumulative plethora of prescriptive codes, conventions, and values. As the person experiences this realm of possibility – namely, the ethical domain – she experiences her action, decision making, and freedom, and thus she ascertains the power of responsibility to proceed with an action. Furthermore, she learns to be more in touch with her inner self as she experiences the undertaking of a moral action. On the other hand, the ethical realm of possibility highlights the limitations and constrictions that are associated with a moral undertaking as one, for instance, accepts the limitations that are interwoven with having a job. The ethical sphere, as a level of possibility, may lead to despondency and despair as it is embedded within a vulnerable system that is subject to failure. It is intrinsically subject to human errors.

The third level of possibility, according to Kierkegaard, happens in the religious sphere where passion, inwardness, truth, fullness, and power demonstrate themselves. The religious stage is a stage where one is deeply engaged with the inner life, a possibility that does not occur for the aesthete or for the ethical. The religious realm of possibility characterizes the most passionate mode of human possibility. The religious sphere of possibility portrays the relationship with God and acknowledgment of eternity. It illustrates the infinite possibilities and its widening horizons. The religious sphere reveals the profound layer of spirituality where one practically experiences being an itinerant of the inner life with passion and faith. The religious sphere is imbued in the personal testimony of the presence of God. The religious sphere relates one to one's infinite potentiality. According to Kierkegaard, the religious sphere provides the realm of possibility where becoming the self is possible, where one needs to be related to oneself, and, more importantly, where one needs to be related to God – that is, the power that creates and constitutes the self.

It is important to note that these levels of possibilities, in Kierkegaard's viewpoint, are not explicating the ways of believing or knowing, and they are not describing the cognitive and epistemological framework of someone. Instead, they are presenting how one is living; thus, they are ontologically defining one's stages of being.

Kierkegaard presents possibility in the same vein and demonstrates how possibilities are infinite in the realm of spirituality. He also posits that the impossibility of possibility can fade away as inwardness opens up room for multitudes of possibilities, even in a world governed by analytical reasoning.

Kierkegaard's critique of Hegelian philosophy and its focus on rationalism propounds the significance of passion instead of reason, with passion opening up the avenues of possibilities. The power of passion and its creational possibilities is characterized in the internal quest for spiritual connectedness and inwardness as Kierkegaard exemplifies Abraham as the hero of faith and possibilities.

Kierkegaard's standpoint on philosophy is uniquely interwoven in the play of passion and practice. He disdains the viewpoint on philosophy that is merely engaged in the abstract conversations of the past. In his book *Either/Or*, Kierkegaard (1959) demonstrates how his philosophy is not in pursuit of the same principles of his contemporary philosophers and indicates,

> The philosopher says, "That's the way it has been hitherto." I ask, "What am I to do if I don't want to become a philosopher?" For if I want to do that, I see clearly enough that I, like the other philosophers, shall soon get to the point of mediating the past.... There is no answer to my questions of

what I ought to do, for if I was the most gifted philosophical mind that ever lived in the world, there must be one more thing I have to do besides sitting and contemplating the past." (pp. 175, 171)

Jung is also among the psychologists who have questioned the material nature of human beings and broadened the spectrum of sensibility, meaning, understanding, and existence. In discussing the relationship between wellness and an immaterial perspective, Jung says,

> During the past thirty years, people from all the civilized countries of the earth have consulted me. Many hundreds of patients have passed through my hands, the greater number being Protestants, a lesser number Jews, and not more than five or six believing Catholics. Among all my patients in the second half of life – that is to say, over thirty-five – there has not been one whose problem in the last resort was not that of finding a religious outlook on life.
>
> It is safe to say that every one of them fell ill, because he had lost what the living religions of every age have given to their followers, and none of them has been really healed who did not regain his religious outlook. This of course has nothing to do with a particular creed or membership of a church. (quoted in Tacey, 2006, pp. 85–86)

Elaborating on Jung's discussion on the unreality of our taken-for-granted reality, which has limited our understanding of human innerness, Tacey (2006) writes,

> Our minds are conditioned to think that only what we can see and touch is real, but Jung questioned this view, and his psychology is a challenge to our understanding of reality. Jung was an unsettling thinker, because he introduced the notion that the evidence of our sense is illusory, and that common sense is nothing more than a construct of external conditioning. (p. 12)

Jung questions and challenges the absolutism of the scientific discourse and its monarchical manifestations in endorsing the validity of the truth through logical positivism and linear forms of thinking. He calls for a genuine search for knowledge and wisdom and opens up the possibility of exploring inspiration and intuition as real modes of knowing and learning. Jung critiques materialism and its implications for humanness:

> We have become rich in knowledge, but poor in wisdom. The centre of gravity of our interest has switched over to the materialistic side, whereas the ancients preferred a move of thought nearer to the fantastic type. To the classical mind, everything was still saturated with mythology. (quoted in Tacey, 2006, p. 15)

In approaching the domain of innerness and explicating a Jungian understanding of the inner world, Tacey (2006) argues that

[w]e tend to think of myths and religions as 'untrue' and of dreams as "distortions of reality." But for Jung they are expressions of a truth that is truer than literal truth.

This is Jung's vital message, linking him to the "perennial philosophy" and to wisdom traditions that originate from Heraclitus, Socrates and Plato. Socrates said truth is not self evident, and Jung would agree. What we see, and what we seem, is not the whole truth. Our knowledge is not reliable; it is partial and undermined by the fact that the unconscious has a separate truth dimension, of which we are mostly oblivious. Ironically, deeper truth resides in what we habitually dismiss as illusion, fantasy, myth and distortion. This may be one reason why, in an age governed by science and logic, our entertainment is saturated with fantasy, mythic stories and legends: a compensatory process has risen in popular culture.

The reason we have lost access to the deeper truth, for Jung, is that we have lost access to the symbolic language that discloses it. Our world-blinded consciousness has made a successful adaptation to external reality, but the cost has been an atrophy of our symbolic life. (p. 15)

Discussing morality, ethics, and wisdom, Kupperman (2005) argues that in order to develop wisdom, one needs to experience a personal transformation. Elucidating the importance of role models in the realization of wisdom, Kupperman (2005, p. 257) explicates the relationship between knowing how to live a good life and a development in the inner sphere and states,

> The wisdom that Buddha regards as crucial follows from the doctrine of anatman (that there is no atman). In the light of this wisdom, desires wither away. If there is no substantial "me" (whether its nature is irreducibly individual or not), desires lose their point. Good (altruistic and compassionate) moral choice naturally follows from this, and wisdom must lead to a sense of what is important in life: a detached, mildly compassionate set of attitudes that includes peacefulness and some inner joy (see Collins, 1982).

Etheredge (2005, p. 308) defines wise policies with eight values for human betterment: power, enlightenment (education and personal growth), wealth, well-being (physical and mental), skill, affection, rectitude, and respect. In doing so, Etheredge highlights the relationship between self and public policy and states that such cultivation of the self in a co-humanity with others was the essential policy foundation of personal health and inner harmony, social order, political stability, good (i.e., righteous and benevolent) government, and universal peace (Creel, 1960; Jaspers, 1962).

Frankl (1967) also focuses on the relationship between meaning and human life and reiterates that human innerness is of great significance in changing one's life through finding one's meaning.

One should point out that parallel, if not similar, assessments of materialist and reductionist science, as well as of the nature and higher purpose of humanity, are equally present in the tradition of Western humanism, albeit from different philosophical and religious standpoints. For example, Martin Heidegger (1999), in his critique of the biologically determined self within the Western discourse of modernism, discussed the pernicious factors that intensify the malaise of modern man and bring about destruction.

Furthermore, Heidegger (1995) contended that the self is entangled within the manacles of materially oriented modernism and experiences emptiness as it goes through pseudo identification with the illusory manifestations of the materialistic world. He argued that we become oblivious to our emptiness in the pervasive discourse of modernism, which is rife with "massiveness, acceleration and calculation" (p. 83).

Our obliviousness engages us in identifying with things that provide us with a superficial sense of comfort and tranquility, but soon they reveal their ostentatiously hollow complexion. Consumerism, competitiveness, emulation, and greed for power and wealth marshal their forces of attraction as the self endlessly follows the slope of emptiness to its abyss. From a psychological standpoint, Cushman (1990) describes the manifold dimensions of emptiness and absence in a materialistic society when he writes that the absent person

> seeks the experience of being continually filled up by consuming goods, calories, experiences, politicians, romantic partners, and empathic therapists in an attempt to combat the growing alienation and fragmentation of its era. [He] is dependent on the continual consumption of nonessential and quickly obsolete items or experiences [...] accomplished through the dual creation of easy credit and a gnawing sense of emptiness in the self. (p. 601)

Cushman (1990) further commented on the emptiness caused by the illusion of abundance created by postmodern consumerism:

> This is a powerful illusion. And what fuels the illusion, what impels the individual into this illusion, is the desperation to fill up the empty self. [...] It must consume in order to be soothed and integrated; it must "take in" and merge with a self-object celebrity, an ideology, or a drug, or it will be in danger of fragmenting into feelings of worthlessness and confusion. (p. 606)

From a different philosophical position, Jürgen Habermas (1973), discerning the dangers of technological entrapment through submission to the manifold presentations of multiplicity, delineated the same ambiguous picture of mainstream scientific reductionism and its worrisome implications.

CHAPTER 7

Heartfulness

It may be safe to say that psychological discussions of peace have been mainly embedded within a mind-oriented approach – notably, a focus on the mind is constantly traceable there. Emphasis on the mind is preponderantly articulated and purported in an array of research, with a focus on well-being, health, development, empowerment, and so forth. Additionally, the mind is conspicuously salient in numerous therapeutic interventions.

To exemplify this, Gilbert's (1991) distinction of Cartesian and Spinozan forms of reality occurs in the context of the mind. Similarly, Epstein's (1998) classification of rational and logical thinking versus experiential and rational thinking is also embedded within a mind-oriented paradigm.

Correspondingly, Sternberg's (2005) discussion of foolishness, its nature, and its taxonomy all takes place in a mind-induced context. Sternberg recounts numerous examples of foolishness demonstrating that being smart is not sufficient to avoid making mistakes. In corroborating his arguments, Sternberg (2005) states,

> Examples of foolish behavior in smart people abound. Bill Clinton, a graduate of Yale Law School and a Rhodes Scholar, compromised his presidency by his poor handling of a scandal involving Monica Lewinsky and other women from his past. More recently, the administration of George W. Bush (who himself was also a Yale graduate) seems to have gotten itself into a war with Iraq in the absence of any preformulated coherent and workable plan for postwar reconstruction and governance. The antics of Silvio Berlusconi, one of the richest men in the world and the prime minister of Italy, at times seem to defy belief (or at least, my own), such as his denial that Mussolini was responsible for any of the deaths of his countrymen but rather only sent some Italians "on vacation." And lest all this seem recent, we only need to go back to Neville Chamberlain and his slogan of "peace in our time" as a means to appease Hitler to realize that smart people can act very foolishly, or so it seems. (pp. 331–332)

On the strength of different works from Grigorenko and Lockery (2002) on heuristics and its relationship with foolish thinking, Austin and Deary (2002) on the relationship between foolish thinking and personality problems, and Moldoveanu and Langer (2002) on the construct of mindlessness as a sign of poor thinking, Sternberg (2005) presents his theory of foolishness in connection with five fallacies. In all these findings, the focus is on the mind, its operation, its categorization, its vulnerabilities, and so forth. To support his arguments on a theory of foolishness where the centerpiece is a mind embroiled with fallacies, Sternberg (2005) writes,

> Take, for example, a corrupt business executive at a company such as Enron, the former monolith that went bankrupt because of mismanagement and corruption. The what-me-worry fallacy is exemplified by the formation and execution of code-named schemes to sequester assets that would have embarrassed all but the most brazen of scamsters. The egocentrism fallacy was exemplified by the executives' demonstration of a complete disregard for anyone but themselves in their unending attempts to enrich themselves at the expense of employees, stockholders, and consumers. The omniscience fallacy was shown by them acting like they had financial acumen and genius that they clearly did not have.
>
> The omnipotence fallacy was shown by their belief that the assets of the corporation were their own personal piggy bank with which they could do whatever they chose. And the invulnerability fallacy was shown by their confidence that they could behave in utterly outrageous ways and not get caught. (p. 338)

All these scholarly works are enterprises that are tied to the mind. The mind has served as the centerpiece for exploring human relationships, human nature, human malaise, human happiness, and human tranquility.

In *Spiritual Evolution: A Scientific Defense of Faith*, Vaillant (2008) presents arguments and evidence to corroborate and substantiate the sensibility of faith and spirituality. Vaillant utilizes a paradigmatic analysis of mainstream reductionist, scientific discourse to prove the very plausibility of faith and spirituality itself – a goal that has been long consigned to oblivion or pushed to the margins by the dominant discourse. Vaillant (2008) indicates that

> [s]keptical academic minds have tended not to accept the universal importance of spirituality in human life.
>
> Too often the mere mention of spirituality leads academics to roll their eyes with the same disbelief – dare I say disgust – with which Skinner treated emotion. Academics have wished to keep scientific and spiritual truths separate, insisting that the scientific truth is truer than the spiritual. I believe that is a mistake. (p. 206)

In continuing his arguments, Vaillant (2008) continues,

> The mistrust that both psychoanalysis and science entertain toward spirituality reminds me of the fable of a miner who was a heavy drinker. He pawned his furniture. He beat his wife. He abused his children. Then, through the efforts of a local priest, he became a fervent member of his local church. Down in the pits his fellow miners ribbed him about "getting religion." One day they asked him if he really believed the miracle of Christ turning water into wine. "I don't understand anything about miracles or how they work," he replied. "I am a simple man. But I do know that in my house liquor has been turned into furniture, despair into hope, and hatred into love. And that's miracle enough for me." Any program that fosters positive emotion is worth taking seriously. Honey catches more flies than vinegar. (p. 205)

Vaillant (2008) quotes historian Karen Armstrong, who suggests,

> The one and only test of a valid religious idea, doctrinal statement, spiritual experience, or devotional practice was that it must lead directly to practical compassion. If your understanding of the divine made you kinder, more empathic, and impelled you to express this sympathy in concrete acts of loving-kindness, this was good theology. But if your notion of God made you unkind, belligerent, cruel, or self-righteous, or if it led you to kill in God's name, it was bad theology. Compassion was the litmus test for the prophets of Israel, for the rabbis of the Talmud, for Jesus, for Paul, and for Muhammad, not to mention Confucius, Lao-tzu, the Buddha. (pp. 205–206)

It is interesting to note that notwithstanding his rigorous arguments in defense of faith and spirituality, Vaillant's system of presentations and substantiation moves in the context of the mainstream psychological viewpoint.

In seeking assistance to demonstrate his statements' plausibility, he refers to Wilson, suggesting, "Once again, sociobiologist Edward O. Wilson comes to our rescue: The essence of humanity's spiritual dilemma is that we evolved genetically to accept one truth and discovered another" (Vaillant, 2008, p. 205).

To solidify his concluding statements, Vaillant (2008) highlights the mainstream terminology and indicates that

> [h]umanity evolved to accept the truth that the highest values of humanity could be expressed through limbic awe for the beautiful and through the enduring guidance of positive emotions. The science that humanity has discovered allows dispassionate reflection in order to validate – and when necessary invalidate – the perceptions of our five senses. Science reflects our

cognitive urge to analyze the world and render it both conscious and predictable. Our task in the future is to integrate Wilson's two truths. For example, a hundred $1 bills are worth more than a hundred love letters. And yet a single love letter is worth more than $100. (p. 205)

In focusing on spiritual emotions, Vaillant (2008) reiterates that

[a]we and the sense of the sacred are dismissed as superstitious and infantile by both the new evolutionary humanists like Daniel Dennett and Richard Dawkins and the older psychoanalytic humanists like Sigmund Freud. Yet awe is the most "spiritual" of the positive emotions. (p. 180)

Along with offering a new paradigm of thinking, other scholars – including some of the existential and humanistic psychologists and existential positive psychologists – have talked about different reference points with distinct features.

Cottinghan (2020) brings a shift of attention and highlights the significance of paying attention to the soul. In elaborating the relationship between the soul and human life, he indicates that

[t]o say we have a soul is partly to say that we humans, despite all our flaws, are fundamentally oriented towards the good. We yearn to rise above the waste and futility that can so easily drag us down and, in the transformative human experiences and practices we call "spiritual," we glimpse something of transcendent value and importance that draws us forward. In responding to this call, we aim to realise our true selves, the selves we were meant to be. This is what the search for the soul amounts to; and it is here, if there is a meaning to human life, that such meaning must be sought.

In defending religious experience as an authentic and genuine experience, Vaillant (2008, p. 80) notes,

Recent studies by Jeffrey Saver and John Rabin have clarified the criteria for distinguishing mystical experiences from insanity. In mystical experiences, visions are usually visual and last for minutes or hours. In paranoid schizophrenia, hallucinations are usually auditory and can last for years. In schizophrenia, the dominant affect is most often terror, and schizophrenic religious delusions are more often associated with omnipotence. In mystical experience, the affect is more often joy and ecstasy, and the individual religious illusions are not of omnipotence but of being a humble servant to a higher power. The language of mystical experience is easily communicated and is socially empathic. The language of schizophrenia is bizarre, eccentric, difficult to understand, and often socially inappropriate. Paul's Second Letter to the Corinthians is pretty straightforward, benign, and easy to understand. The Revelation to John is bizarre, terrifying, and to many incomprehensible. (p. 80)

Jung discusses the importance of the invisible "I" and the spiritual and transcendental self for growth, development, health, wellness, and inner calmness and considers the path to the transcendental realm as a constructive step toward one's well-being. Along with Jung's emphasis on the hero's journey, Campbell (1949/ 2008) iterates that

> [a] hero ventures forth from the world of common day into a region of supernatural wonder: fabulous forces are there encountered and a decisive victory is won: the hero comes back from this mysterious adventure with the power to bestow boons on his fellow man. (p. 23)

The use of a different language has bespoken the possibility of going beyond the materialist way of looking at existence and has considered meaning as one of the vital elements of human relatedness to the realm of the invisible.

Correspondingly, an alternative concentration has loomed in the overblown domain of mind-induced predilections with a focus on heart. To so many, heart may be associated with emotion, passion, fervor, and enthusiasm. To a number of others, heart may be linked to the physiological heart. When used metaphorically, distinctly and independent from the bodily oriented heart, the meaning of heart has demonstrated an expansive, rich repertoire of allusions and attributions, as well as an elucidation on an essence that may be unbeknownst to those afflicted with a mundane connotation of heart.

Explicating Emerson's words on "the world's hearts," Solomon, Marshall, and Gardner (2005) argue,

> In a famous 1837 address, Ralph Waldo Emerson exhorted "professionals" – including the "American scholars" of his audience – to undertake their work wisely. By this, Emerson meant looking beyond both remote matters and minutiae to become "the world's eye" and "the world's heart." Such professionals should "resist the vulgar prosperity that retrogrades ever to barbarism, by preserving and communicating heroic sentiments, noble biographies, melodious verse, and the conclusions of history." In today's world, Emerson's call for professionals to aspire to the lofty goal of societal stewardship is likely to sound both naive and decidedly out of character with the nature of contemporary professions. After all, the professions of the early 21st century – medicine, accounting, law, and the like – are beset by unprecedented economic, ethical, and technological challenges that were unimaginable in Emerson's day. (p. 272)

In line with the perception of heart as a physical organ, some, including Sardello (2006), have developed a link between the heart as a physiological entity and the spiritual heart. Sardello focuses on the nature of the heart and argues that "it functions simultaneously as a physical, psychic, and spiritual organ" (p. 82).

Sardello (2006, p. 86) calls for an exploration of the physical heart – its chambers, its dynamics – and suggests that activating our sensations in close physical contacts with the heart will take us to perceive "pure intimacy . . . intimacy without something or someone attached to that intimacy." Coming from a phenomenological psychology, Sardello (2006) describes the nature of the physical heart as "inherently spiritual" and argues that the inherent activity of the heart is essentially a spiritual activity.

In keeping with understanding the heart beyond the mechanical tool that operates merely as a pumping apparatus, Pearce (2002, pp. 64–65) indicates that "the heart takes on the subtle individual colors of a person without losing its essential universality. It seems to mediate between our individual self and a universal process while being representative of that universal process."

Interestingly enough, the traditional texts go beyond the physiological meaning of heart and discuss heart as the key to spirituality, transcendence, salvation, emancipation, and liberation. The following words are from Jesus concerning the Beatitudes in the Bible (Matthew 5:8): "Blessed are the pure in heart, for they shall see God." Other examples include the following in Ezekiel:

> I will take you from the nations and gather you from all the countries, and bring you into your own land. I will sprinkle clean water upon you, and you shall be clean from all your uncleannesses, and from all your idols I will cleanse you. A new heart I will give you, and a new spirit I will put within you; and I will remove from your body the heart of stone and give you a heart of flesh. I will put my spirit within you and make you follow my statutes and be careful to observe my ordinances. Then you shall live in the land I gave to your ancestors, and you shall be my people and I will be your God. (Ezekiel 36:24–28)

Along parallel lines, orthodox texts highlight the significance of the heart in its spiritual stance, stating,

> When we read in the writings of the Fathers about the place of the heart which the mind finds by way of prayer, we must understand by this the spiritual faculty that exists in the heart. Placed by the creator in the upper part of the heart, this spiritual faculty distinguishes the human heart from the heart of animals. . . .
>
> The intellectual faculty in man's soul, though spiritual, dwells in the brain, that is to say in the head: in the same way, the spiritual faculty which we term the spirit of man, though spiritual, dwells in the upper part of the

> heart, close to the left nipple of the chest and a little above it.
> (Kadloubovsky & Palmer, 1966, p. 190)

Or consider the following:

> To stand guard over the heart, to stand with the mind in the heart, to
> descend from the head to the heart – all these are one and the same thing.
> The core of the work lies in concentrating the attention and the standing
> before the invisible Lord, not in the head but in the chest, close to the heart
> and in the heart. When the divine warmth comes, all this will be clear.
> (Kadloubovsky & Palmer, 1966, p. 194)

Presenting the most delicate human feelings in his world-renowned
poetic fable *The Little Prince*, Antoine de Saint-Exupéry (1943, p. 68)
elucidates the vitality of the heart in the language of the fox when the fox
says, "It is only with the heart that one can see rightly; what is essential is
invisible to the eye."

In discussing the distance between mainstream psychology and many of
its forgotten enterprises, Schneider (1998) refers to Frank Farley's speech
to the APA and says,

> When the 1994 president of the American Psychological Association, Frank
> Farley, suggested that we psychologists "stand very close to being a discipline
> concerned with superficial problems" and that spirituality, "deep feelings
> about soul and eternity ... [and] a psychology of meaning in the broadest
> sense ... placing the mystery of life in context, and most importantly,
> showing the road to generosity and love" will "become increasingly impor-
> tant" (cited in Martin, 1994, p. 12), he was sounding a romantic chord.

Relative to understanding the subtlety of the human soul, Schneider
focuses on romantic psychology and indicates that although marginal in its
influence, romanticism has a long and distinguished lineage in psychology.
Romantic psychology faces a grave diminution of its influence. This
development is based in part on the shortcomings of romanticism itself,
but it is also in large part due to converging political, economic, and
professional interests.

Explicating the necessity of paying attention to a psychology that
addresses the delicacies of humanness, Schneider (1998) expounds how
negligence toward psychological understanding of romanticism has
brought us irreparable damages, stating,

> There is a formidable price to be paid for the eroding of romanticism's
> influence in psychology. This price includes psychology's deepening neglect
> of its meaning and significance for the lifeworld; its further dissociation
> from the arts and humanities; and its widening reductionism.

Schneider calls for celebrating a postmodern, neoromantic psychology that may give rise to alternative ways of looking at the human soul beyond the reductionist models of mainstream psychology. These are models that too often confine human beings to mechanical configurations. In doing so, Schneider (1998) says,

> Is it beyond the present imagination to conceive of a romantic revival in psychology? Perhaps. At the very least, however, the romantic psychology that I have been discussing compels significantly more attention than it has heretofore garnered or is currently receiving. Although the kind of romantic revolution that I urge in this article (and that others have urged elsewhere) is far-reaching, and the resources necessary to meet it are formidable, psychologists, from my standpoint, would be remiss to overlook it. The real question is whether we as a profession are going to act in an expedient way – in conformity with fashionable trends – or in accord with our professional mandate? If no one stands up for principle (as opposed to fashion) in our field there will surely be few capable of taking this stance in our stead. Even if one is a tough-minded empiricist, one must recognize our field's multidimensionality. One must recognize that psychology cannot simply stand for a monolithic curriculum or one-track science (Koch, 1993; Rychlak, 1993). It must open to the larger view of science embodied by a growing constituency, the view supported in many cases by clinicians but that relates to the field as a whole: that is, the view of psychology as a human inquiry, one tailored to people's lived realities. As the early romanticists taught, such a view may well help to salvage our planet as well as our discipline. (pp. 286–287)

Speaking of the heart's consciousness, Sardello (2006) says,

> When we engage in the practices of Silence, we are going to the heart's consciousness. We practice living within the activity of feeling, not the activity of having feelings but of locating the center of our consciousness within feeling. Heart consciousness and feeling are equivalent to each other. In usual consciousness, feeling is more vague than the clarity of thinking, but in heart awareness this is reversed. Feeling becomes intense and clear, while the cognition that is present does not dominate. We come to these revelations concerning the heart and Silence not by theorizing but from the immediacy of experiencing. It is possible to develop the consciousness of the heart. In doing so, we are able to enter into a remarkable intensity of Silence and become aware in a far more concentrated manner of the creativity, the healing, the devotion, and all the other qualities of Silence spoken of thus far. Through practices of the heart we become not just partakers of the gifts of Silence but also spiritual creators within this realm. We approach this awesome possibility with greatest reverence and humility for it is a creating act of our soul-spirit rather than an attempt to use the Silence of the heart to make something happen. Entering into the heart is a practice of entering the miraculous. (p. 95)

In his book *Living Presence: A Sufi Guide to Mindfulness and the Essential Self*, Helminski (1992, pp. 157, 158) explores the nature of heart in Islamic mysticism and says,

> We have subtle subconscious faculties we are not using. Beyond the limited analytic intellect is a vast realm of mind that includes psychic and extrasensory abilities; intuition; wisdom; a sense of unity; aesthetic, qualitative and creative faculties; and image-forming and symbolic capacities. Though these faculties are many, we give them a single name with some justification for they are working best when they are in concert. They comprise a mind, moreover, in spontaneous connection to the cosmic mind. This total mind we call "heart."
>
> The heart is the antenna that receives the emanations of subtler levels of existence. The human heart has its proper field of function beyond the limits of the superficial, reactive ego-self. Awakening the heart, or the spiritualized mind, is an unlimited process of making the mind more sensitive, focused, energized, subtle, and refined, of joining it to its cosmic milieu, the infinity of love.

Further explicating the functions of the heart, Helminski (1992, p. 157) adds,

> The heart includes subtle faculties that are beyond the intellect, but as long as we are alive and embodied in physical form, the intellect is a primary interpreter of our experience. The intellect transforms the subtle perceptions of the psyche into recognizable, familiar images and thoughts. It may give the final expression of these faculties, acting as translator and analyzer, but nothing originates with the intellect alone; it rearranges known elements, categorizes, and compares. Sometimes it does this in an elegant and purposeful way; other times it makes false connections, or reduces new information to old concepts, functioning in a mechanical, habitual manner. The art of intuitive living depends on the ability to accurately translate subtle perceptions as they emerge from the subconscious into consciousness.

In discussing the distinct status of the heart and its unique realm, Rumi states,

> So, the heart will be as a substance and the world like an accident. How can the shadow of the heart meet the needs of the heart? Delineating the function of the heart, John Keats says: I am certain of nothing but the Heart's affections and the truth of the Imagination.

In addition to sundry manifestations of the locutionary application of heart in a wide variety of religious and mystical texts, I want to present, propose, and propound another view of heart that may be mostly unknown to Western readers. As is often also the case with Western humanism vis-à-vis

Christian dogma and the life and teachings of Jesus Christ, discussions of various Islamic perspectives on humanistic issues, including philosophical and religious ones, may concentrate on texts and documents that, albeit Islamic, reflect the ideas, doctrines, and viewpoints of individual Muslim scholars and not necessarily what is inherited from Prophet Mohammad, his manners, his Household, Hadith, and the Quran.

Although the ideas and perspectives of different Muslim scholars may provide information on the given topics, they may also be reflective and representative of the specific historical and cultural contexts that they have been exposed to. For example, the Muslim scholars who, through the translation of Greek peripatetic texts, were inspired to ponder the implications of these texts for the Islamic school of thought were ultimately embedded within a domain that demonstrated their own intellectual creativity and not necessarily the Islamic viewpoints inherited from the Prophet Mohammad, the Quran, or the Prophet's Household.

This situation is even traceable in the citations of numerous Muslim scholars who have acknowledged the distinction between the creative discourses resulting from the interplay of their own cogitations and the pure Islam of Prophet Mohammad. To give just one example, one may cite Ibn Sina, known as Avicenna (AD 980–1037), when he questions the comprehensiveness and impeccability of the human intellect:

> It is not in the capacity of human beings to apprehend the truth of things. We merely apprehend the accidental features and the formal characteristics of things without apprehending the true nature of things and their real distinguishing features. Our understanding provides us with the discernment that there are things in the world with their characteristics and features. Nonetheless, the true nature of the primordial source, the intellect, the soul, the fire, the celestial bodies, the water and the earth are unknown to us. We cannot even grasp the accidental (A'raz) features of the things. (Avicenna, Hijri 1404)

In other numerous works, including the Treatise on Definitions (*Resalate Alhodood*) and the Book of Debates (*Almobahesat*), Avicenna ascertained the limitations of the human-made intellect and its circumscribing implications. (Avicenna, Hijri 1404, pp. 34–35).

The same idea can be found in the works of other scholars such as Khaje Nasseereddine Toosee, who shows the inability and incompetency of human intellect in apprehending the true nature of things, illustrating, at the same time, the urgent and striking need of the human intellect for divine revelation and revealed inspiration. He clearly indicated that "intellect cannot lead to what the prophets instruct" (Noorani, 1980, p. 53).

Sheikh Alla Addin Toosee, in reiterating the feebleness of the human intellect, indicated that it alone "cannot grasp the truths behind the issues of theology, and the philosophical and intellectual ideas and doctrines cannot substantiate the consummate apprehension of these issues without the confirmation and support from the source of revelation namely God" (Azzakheere, as cited by Hakimi, 1997, p. 21).

In line with this principle, Shahabeddin Sohrevardee (1355, in Hakimi, 2013) also questioned the possibility of providing a comprehensively impeccable definition for anything, as argued by the peripatetic philosophers. Sadrolmotaaleheen, the great philosopher of Islam, propounded that "even the gifted scholars fail to apprehend the heavenly and earthly truths" (Asfar, as cited by Hakimi, 1997, p. 20). Such words and statements may vividly present the Muslim scholars' confirmation of the inability of the human intellect and the dangers behind what Hakimi (1997, p. 26) calls the "overgeneralization of the domain of intellect." This is not to deny, however, that the very Muslim scholars who have declared the incompetency of the intellect have also rendered huge services through their own contemplative efforts, by virtue of the self-same feeble instrument of their scholarly activities, namely, their reasoning intellect. For example, in reiterating the significant share held by Muslim scholars in shaping the primordial pillars of modern science, Bernal (1954, p. 196) indicated that "it is difficult to estimate the value of the actual contributions to this fund of learning that were provided by Islamic scholars themselves." Explicating the impact of Islam in new inventions and the creation of new modes of knowledge, Bernal added that "Islam became the focal point of Asian and European knowledge. As a result, there came into the common pool a new series of inventions quite unknown and inaccessible to Greek and Roman technology" (p. 195).

The point here is that many prominent Muslim scholars have often drawn a distinction between the reasoning human intellect and the revelation-oriented (*Vahy*) intellect, considering the former to be inferior to the latter. Therefore, although Muslim scholars have contributed to the advancement of knowledge and technology, one needs to make a distinction between the notions, ideas, doctrines, and perspectives presented within the scope of Muslim erudition, on the one hand, and the direct words, instructions, and Hadith of Prophet Mohammad, his Household, and the Quran, on the other hand. Furthermore, Muslim scholars and philosophers themselves, including Mulla Sadra, Ibn Sina, Suhrawardi, and Khajenassereddin Toosee, have frequently acknowledged the necessity of going beyond the human intellect and searching for answers within the sources of revelation, thus questioning the sovereignty of human knowledge in providing comprehensive responses to everything, including the questions of humanism. To exemplify this, Mulla Sadra cited a Hadith from the Prophet Mohammad and instructed, "my friend, explore this Hadith in order to grasp the substance of the knowing about the soul" (in Hakimi, 1997, p. 205).

I have insisted on the distinction between intellectual reasoning and revelation-based intellect because it can help us excavate the ontological, epistemological, and etiological layers of Islamic psychology and its humanism more clearly. Islam, etymologically speaking, comes from the word *Silm*, which means "peace." Islamic "peace" entails diverse human domains, from the intrapersonal relationship to interpersonal communication, international relations, and international negotiations.

The root word of Islam also goes back to *Tasleem*, which literally means "submission and resignation." Imam Ali of Shia (Hakimi, 1997) indicated that Islam consists of submission to any form of truth, thus emphasizing the spirit of openness toward learning, listening, and accepting any manifestation that unveils the complexion of truth in any aspect.

Islam-oriented peace begins with an in-depth understanding of the significance of its ontological perspective, as this ontological layer leads the discourse of human interaction on diverse points. At the core of the Islamic ontological perspective, prevailing interpretations of a human being as a biological animal are nullified. Man is not confined within biological and evolutionary boundaries – a physiological machine that operates at the mercy of purely physiological and biological stimuli. Rather, according to Islam, the underlying spiritual ontology of humankind engenders etiological scopes that can define values beyond the utilitarian hegemony of the biologically driven mandates.

Prophet Mohammad introduced peace and mercy as the essence of relationship management. The Prophet is himself presented by the Quran and numerous Hadiths as the mercy for the world (*Rahmaton lel alameen*). The Quran describes the etiological mission of the Prophet and his ordainment as the completion and consummation of the best possible moral values.

The emphasis on values within the context of the Islamic intercultural perspective suggests that there are unchangeable, universal, and unquestionably valid values that cannot be compromised. "We did not send you except as a mercy to the mankind and the world" (Anbeeya, verse 110).

An Islamic perspective on psychology shows that the mainstream scientific discourse of modernization is embedded within the promotion of multiplicities, fragmentation, and absence: humans are multiplied through the interplay of technologically imposed relationships precisely because they are divided in so many pieces and fragments. As they go about their multifarious tasks, they become so engaged in fragmentation and division that they can no longer experience unity and presence. From an Islamic perspective, psychological humanism, inspired by a utilitarian vision, cannot herald the promise of establishing sustainable human ties, as it is intrinsically planted in a predilection that excludes a quintessential examination of human needs and demands beyond the utilitarian domain.

There is a need to relate to others for persons to flourish, and this may mean valuing others (including the Divine Other) beyond one's own utilitarian drives and consumptive motives. An absence-centered philosophy cannot offer the panacea of presence because it is paralyzed by elements and components that reduce the vitality of being to an indulgence in the frequency of multiplicities.

An Islamic psychological perspective advocates the necessity of presence through revisiting the reference points that have validated our subscription to engaging utilitarian multiplicities. This would presuppose a shift, from a focus on possessiveness to one on Tasleem, to letting go or releasing things.

Power, wealth, paraphernalia, political games, parochialism, egoism, egotism, hubris, arrogance, and imperialism belong to the domain of possessiveness and ineluctably encourage and foster multiplicities. Tasleem, however, promotes the principle of being as the fountain through which togetherness and belonging unfold themselves. From a Quranic perspective, the sublimity of man is verified not through the possession of ephemeral belongings but by virtue of piety and righteousness, or to use the exact Quranic term, *Taqwa*.

It is through the indiscriminate immersion in the world and its engaging multiplicities that Islam argues that human beings experience subjugation and entanglement in shadows and fragmentation, thereby distancing themselves from presence. As people's exposure to multiplicities increases, their degrees of absence multiply, and, through the heightened form of absence, they seek their manifestation in the illusory sedimentations of possessiveness.

Taqwa, however, gives rise to a progressive and proactive form of being and becoming, as it nullifies any form of superiority based on worldly possessiveness such as race, color, and even knowledge. Knowing, if not connected to the fountain of presence, turns out to be a cause of absence; it contributes to the accumulation of masks, disguises, and pretenses.

An absence-driven knowledge gives rise to slavery, control, manipulation, coercion, and aggressiveness. Islamic Hadith from the Prophet Mohammad and his Household frequently reprimand the formation of knowledge that is confined within the borders of egoism.

An absence-driven knowledge cannot augur the possibility of a global intercultural perspective, as it is already enmeshed in the manacles of multiplicities that dictate fixation within the realm of materialism.

A psychological perspective on peace, therefore, needs to address the epistemological and ontological questions of humankind. Much of Western humanistic psychology sees persons as valued because they are deemed valuable, with this worth being self-imposed and not derived from something greater than the material world. The Islamic view goes beyond the animalistic interpretation of human beings. Highlighting the significance of such underlying questions, Nasr (2007) says,

> The evolutionary view of man as animal, which even from the biological point of view is open to question, can tell us little as to the real nature of man; no more than can the theories of many anthropologists who discuss anthropology without even knowing who man, the anthropos, is and without realizing the complete states of universal existence which man carries with him here and now. (p. 69)

The Islamic psychological perspective on peace departs from the utilitarian interpretation of humanity and critiques the approaches and policies that tend to keep humans within the confines of materialism. Deep within the ontological and epistemological perspective on Islamic psychology, there lies an emphasis on the revelation-inspired intellect, which is in pursuit of unity, togetherness, oneness, and presence. Conversely, utilitarian-driven rationalism has its quest for multiplicity, materialism, consumerism, subjugation, exploitation, and absence.

The practical implications of each doctrine would engender diametrically different consequences. The former considers its mission to look for factors that liberate man from the quagmires of stagnation and slavery; it argues that slavery in our world today is not epitomized in the traditionally recognized modes and appearances.

Modern slavery imposes diverse points of illusion and involves numerous forms of disguise. It is shrouded in the pretentious masks of progressiveness, development, and betterment but etiologically looks for domination, mastery, and conquest. It monopolizes, through sundry psychological games, the avenues of understanding and knowing, and limits the possibility of going beyond the preestablished discourse of legitimacy as planted and prescribed by the hegemony of utilitarian rationalism.

The Islamic psychological perspective on peace challenges the confinement of human beings within the borders of egoism and the mundane discourse of consumerism. An Islamic view claims that the world is merely a bridge for growth and development; one cannot linger in a temporary abode, namely, the bridge. Death is just the commencement of eternal life. One needs to be mindful of one's intrapersonal and interpersonal transactions and interactions, as one dwells in the hospice of the world. It behooves humankind, according to the Islamic perspective, to be liberated from the prisons of predilections and suggestions that dictate multifarious forms of slavery and submission. In a Hadith, Imam Sadegh (Hakimi, 1997), the sixth Imam of Shias, pinpointed that people, upon departing this world, may leave as slaves or as liberated beings (*ahrar*).

The Persian poet Rumi, in elucidating the lofty status of humans and their invaluable position in the world, said as follows:

> Wine in ferment is a beggar suing for our ferment;
> Heaven in revolution is a beggar suing for our consciousness;
> Wine was intoxicated with us, not we with it;
> The body came into being from us, not we from it.
>   (cited in Hakimi, 1997, p. 144)

The self, in the materialistic context, is subjugated to sporadic engagements with a monolithic concentration on nothing except the satiation of the ego. The inflation of the ego and its consummation through the hedonistic propensities of the material world will produce alienation, loneliness, separation, and bitterness. It cannot extend a genuine invitation for relationship and togetherness, except as it serves its own needs. The self fails to mobilize the possibility of shared understanding because the spirit of listening ceases to operate when the gates of egoism can only allow the entrance of propositions that comply with preestablished legitimate discourses. Respectful listening fades away when the tyranny of the utilitarian, competitive enterprise expands its ramifications; the possibility of sensibility of the other diminishes under the yoke of ego-driven rationalism.

An Islamic psychological perspective on peace propounds a salient role for consciousness, understanding, contemplation, awareness, and wisdom. A Hadith from Imam Sadegh (Babeveyh, 1983) indicates that for anyone whose two days (in living and understanding) are equal, he or she is at a loss.

In another narrative, Imam Ali, addressing Komyel, one of his companions, said, "Beware that you are in dire need of contemplation in any move, albeit small or minor" (Harrani, 1984, p. 171). Jafari (2004) demonstrated that there are at least 40 verses in the Quran that call for contemplation, thoughtfulness, and wisdom.

An Islamic psychological view on peace focuses on relationship aware- ness and management, along with management of interdependencies, as the pillars of interconnected networks of humanity.

In a Hadith cited from Imam Reza (Hakimi, 1997), the eighth Imam of Shias, half of wisdom is characterized through the practical demonstration of kindness and compassion toward people. In a series of similar Hadith from the Prophet and his Household (Hakimi, Hakimi, & Hakimi, 2005), the key to societal management lies in relationship management and the accurate understanding of management interdependencies. A profound exploration of Quranic verses and Hadith along with the Sireh (behavior and communication) of the Prophet shows Islam's great emphasis on the significance of relationship, its management, and its implications.

Monotheism (*Tawhid*) as the first and foremost principle of Islam unfolds itself not only as a philosophical principle but also as a source of inspiration for relationship management in diverse human transactions. Monotheism enriches one's security as one's fear and anxiety are left behind through a transcendental process of self-exploration and the attain- ment of faith in God's oneness and that as a place to relate to others.

This process may be clearly traceable in the cooperative spirit of Muslims in the early years of Islam's emergence as they pioneered the transmission of science and knowledge. For example, at the beginning of the third century (Hijri calendar), there were 80 Muslim academic faculties and departments in Spain (Jafari, 2004).

Through a shift from the external manifestations of security to the internal source of security, Muslims were inspired by the Prophet to overcome seemingly insurmountable difficulties and challenges – monotheism became the panacea for managing both intrapersonal and interpersonal relationships.

Prayer was considered the elevation and ascension of humankind, as it opened up a new chapter for relationships between the self and the Creator. Islamic relationship awareness may offer a turning point in understanding intercultural humanism within Islamic psychology because it introduces the connectedness of all human beings in a large cosmological project where all are linked to the Creator.

The problem in our world today, according to Islam, lies in the degeneration of values as a result of egoism and egotism. Values are no longer taken as ends but means, in a limited spectrum at that, with limited application. This can contribute to a distance from heartfulness.

The Islamic psychological perspective on peace propounds that for as long as we do not revive shared human values, through which humanity gains its decency, we will be merely pretending to elaborate emancipative discourses for humanity, which are in fact disconnected from the living reality.

It is in line with this understanding of the role of values in our being and becoming that Islam considers the revitalization of one human being as the revitalization of all human beings, and the killing of one human being as the killing of all human beings. The Quran explicitly makes this point (Ch. Ma'edde, verse 32). Furthermore, Quranic verses along with a wide array of Hadiths from the Prophet and his Household call for mindful and consistent implementation of these values in practice. The Quran reprimands those who instruct others to follow virtue and piety but who themselves do not practice what they preach. In a Hadith from Imam Sadegh of Shias (Hakimi et al., 2005), he points out that Muslims need to show the path to monotheism and virtue through their deeds and actions, not through their words.

Authentic human values, according to Islam, cannot be taken seriously and cannot be put into effect except through a quest for meaning and its connectedness to the Creator. If life is nothing except pleasure in the ephemeral earthly abode and its associated desires, then it cannot give rise to a genuine source of care for others.

The "Other" is, in a materialist perspective, translated in the body of the earthly desires and their ramifications. "Others" make sense as long as they move in line with the manifestations of solipsism, egoism, egotism, and self-satisfying interests. Yes, attention to the "Others" can also be meaningful if negligence toward them would hurt self-centered concentration – but, there is no sense of togetherness, no true care for others.

An Islamic psychological perspective moves in the completely opposite direction: any extension, manifestation, and crystallization of being is revered and respected as they all unveil their being signs from God. In an instruction to Maleke Ashtar (Jafari, 2004), his newly appointed governor-general, Imam Ali, the first Imam of Shias, urged him to appreciate the subtlety of the rights of the people. He instructed him that when one is with people, one must make sure to share eye contact with everyone present, and not only with the privileged.

One should also be mindful of other people's rights and values, Imam Ali advised Maleke, even if one happens to encounter people who do not abide by one's own values and viewpoints. You should not impose your views on them or act differently toward them because they are, if nothing else, endowed with the gift of being from God; they are created by God, and they should be revered as his creations (Razee, 1993, pp. 427–445).

Any sense of inferiority or superiority dissipates in the context of Islam's monotheistic perspective. Wealth, power, position, and possessions cannot offer a sense of true elevation; neither can they confer any social status. Thus, an Islamic perspective on peace underlines the significance of social justice as a universal human value because justice is considered, according to the Quran, one of the main missions of all the prophets. Without justice, there will be no living sense of values because if justice perishes, it gives way to the growth of a wide variety of malaise, promoting hypocrisy, manipulation, exploitation, and abuse (Hakimi, 1997).

Prophets were ordained to provide people with relationship management in four different spectra: (a) intrapersonal relationship, (b) interpersonal relationship, (c) relationship with nature, and (d) relationship with God. A self entrapped in egoism, greed, and possessiveness is overwhelmed by an ever-increasing flux of attention toward material reality, the world as it appears in the physical objects, and their earthly invitations. Such tyranny fails to see the quintessential complexion of humanity, as it is blinded by a monolithic parochialism that merely prescribes the accumulation of self-inflated objectives.

Intrapersonal mismanagement, according to Islam, has largely contributed to the expansion of corruption and the devastation of human relationships in innumerable domains. The roots of severe pollution and malaise in our world today, from environmental pollution to the massacre of human beings, are found in misdirected self-management or lack of self-management.

How can effective self-management operate in an interpersonal relationship when the self is already at the mercy of ruining forces that dictate sole obedience to the infinite waves of the inflation-seeking self? A self inflated by hubris, superiority, and arrogance is too entrenched in the basin of self-centeredness to be able to look at the circumferences of the other.

The Islamic perspective on peace indicates that self-management ought to have the highest priority of any pedagogical agenda, as it is through the demolished sense of self-elevation that the agony of oppression, discrimination, injustice, poverty, and other human-made catastrophes transpire. The sense of elevation and transcendence cannot happen for the self within itself because the self is, ipso facto, in dire need of connectedness, belonging, attachment, and dependencies. The self is, essentially, inadequate to engender the required efficacy of management because it is constantly threatened and deceived by the forces that maintain to support it but are merely in pursuit of its interests within the scope of the body.

Monotheism (*Tawhid*) begins with understanding the nothingness of anything except God. This nothingness acknowledges that anything in the realm of existence is nothing except through a connection to God. Once the connectedness of things is negated, their being is negated. Analogically speaking, beings operate as prepositional modes: a preposition loses its sense of being the moment it is placed outside a sentence. Ontologically, beings are beings as long as they are connected to God, or Allah, to borrow the Arabic word.

To address the arguments of those who might see the forgoing statements as contravening the notion of vice (*shar*), the Muslim scholars, inspired by the Quran and the Hadith, have argued that vice, or any of its manifestations, does not belong to the realm of *Wujud* (existence) because it falls into the category of nonexistence; for instance, ignorance is nothing except the lack of knowledge, as oppression consists in nothing save the absence of justice. Vice does not fall into the category of *Wujud* because existence as given by God is epitomized as good.

The monotheistic perspective of Islamic psychology on peace, therefore, concentrates on togetherness, connectedness, and belonging to humanity. The Persian poet Sa'di illustrated this sense of belonging when he depicted the universality of pain that is human in nature: "My complexion did not turn pale because of my own destitution; the sorrow of the destitution of others brought the paleness to me" (Sa'di, 1998, p. 27).

In elaborating the implications of Islamic monotheism for peace, Nasr (2007) wrote,

> It is this basic nature of man which makes a secular and agnostic humanism impossible. It is not metaphysically possible to kill the gods and seek to efface the imprint of the Divinity upon man without destroying man himself; the bitter experience of the modern world stands as overwhelming evidence to this truth. The face which God has turned toward the cosmos and man (the wajh Allah of the Quran) is none other than the face of man toward the Divinity and in fact the human face itself. One cannot "efface" the "face of God" without "effacing" man himself and reducing him to a faceless entity lost in an anthill. The cry of Nietzsche that "God is dead" could not but mean that "man is dead," as the history of the 20th century has succeeded in demonstrating in so many ways. But in reality the response to Nietzsche was not the death of man as such but the Promethean man who had thought he could live on a circle without a center. The other man, the pontifical man, although forgotten in the modern world, continues to live even within those human beings who

pride themselves in having outgrown the models and modes of thought of their ancestors; he continues to live and will never die. (p. 186)

An Islamic psychological perspective on peace does not go with reductionist approaches toward culture and cultural understanding, such as is the case within the discourse of contemporary cultural psychology that, albeit different from the mainstream positivist psychology on the surface, is yet embedded within the same methodological and paradigmatic hegemony (Teo, 2005). Western mainstream psychology is more embedded within the perspective of the observer and not the perspective of the actor. This has led to marginalization, trivialization, and dehumanization of the actors (Fatemi, 2016).

At the center of the Islamic perspective on peace, there lies the solution of love. There are tens of Hadith from the Prophet and his Household that promote the expansion and implementation of love in diverse points of human relationship (e.g., "Half of wisdom lies in kindness and compassion towards people" [Imam Reza] and "Get yourself obliged towards loving all people [Imam Ali, both cited in Hakimi et al., 2005]). Love constitutes the essence of interaction, and it is through love and its manifestations that human transformations occur.

Rumi, the Persian poet, frequently discussed compassion, kindness, and love toward others as the keys of development, change, and transformation. He considered kindness toward others as the answer for human development when he indicated that "kindness changes thorns into flowers, kindness changes the prison into garden. Without kindness and love, garden changes into a place of thorn" (in Jafari, 1995, p. 146).

Liveliness, according to Islamic psychology, is embedded in love and kindness toward others. In a famous Hadith, cited in Amali by Sadoogh (in Hakimi et al., 2005), Imam Ali of Shias reiterated to all Muslims, "let the practice of mercy, forgiveness and kindness towards others be well embedded in your heart" (Hakimi et al., 2005, p. 102).

Portraying the splendor and glory of love, Shariati, an Iranian Muslim sociologist and thinker (1988), describes his pilgrimage to Mecca in the following way:

> As you circumambulate and move closer to the Ka'ba . . . you are a new part of the people.. . . The Ka'ba is the world's sun whose face attracts you into its orbit.. . . You have been transformed into a particle that is gradually melting and disappearing. This is absolute love at its peak. (pp. 54–56)

In his government policies, Imam Ali told his governor-general, Malek Ashtar, that he should "observe and practice kindness, mercy, compassion and respect to anyone in the world because people fall into two groups: They either belong to your Islamic viewpoint and thus they are your companions, or, even if not, they are equal to you in terms of being a human being" (Razee, 1993, p. 427). Imam Reza, the eighth Imam of Shias, also known as the Imam of Mercy (Al Iamam Ar Raoof), considered kindness toward others as half of wisdom. In a famous Hadith from Imam Hossein, the grandson of the Prophet Mohammad and the son of Imam Ali, namely, the fourth Imam of Shias, sins dissipate as one practices being kind toward others (all cited in Hakimi et al., 2005). Referring to the ontological layers of the components of love, Nasr (2007) observed,

> Hence, the love of God and by God permeates the whole universe, and many Islamic mystics or Sufis over the ages have spoken of that love to which Dante refers at the end of the Divine Comedy when he speaks of "the love that moves the sun and the stars." (p. 48)

Love, of course, is focused on the loved one – even if there is a cost to oneself. Such love to God (Allah) and others does not flow from a humanistic view of generic love to all in the world, whereas in reality the desires rooted in love of self may conflict with love of the other.

One does not need to delve too deeply into the repertoire of Islamic perspectives to see the groundlessness of the accusations leveled against Islam in our world today. The misrepresentation of Islam by those who, wittingly or unwittingly, introduce it in the context of terror, aggression, war, bellicosity, and violence is in deep contradiction with the teachings of the Quran, the Prophet Mohammed, and his Household.

Numerous verses in the Quran dignify the quintessential love for human beings apparent in Islam and strongly recommend practicing a loving and caring attitude toward others. This is also obvious in many Islamic prayers, where praying for your fellow worshippers and others is highly recommended. Imam Hassan, the son of Imam Ali and the third Imam of Shias, recalled his mother, Hazrat Zahra, the daughter of Prophet Mohammad, in the time of her nocturnal praying:

> I listened to my mother as she was praying in the middle of the night recounting the names of all neighbors and others in her prayer; and I listened closely and realized that all her prayers were brim with attention toward others and devoid of any concentration on her own person. (Babeveyh, 2007, p. 181)

Islamic psychology refutes the idea of a humanism based on egoism, disguised with pretentiously bombastic names and titles; it calls for an understanding of human bondage beyond race, color, land, position, possessions, or any material ties that may impede the process of implementing a genuine interconnectedness.

Attention toward human bonds and connectedness does not come out of a sentimental predilection toward a people-pleasing attitude in the context of self-satiating needs, but it gains its sensibility and application in the body of the values within Islamic monotheism (*Tawhid*), where respect and attention toward others are presented as values that unfold their significance in the complexion of a monotheist (*Movahhed*).

An Islam-based psychological perspective on peace departs from the materialistic interpretation of human beings, affirms the spiritual component, and considers the path to spirituality as an essential element of growth and development. Humans are created to go beyond the material domain of life, to leap beyond the earthly and instinctual belongings and attachments. The physical, material world is only a passage. An attachment to the material world and its manifestations is like falling in love with the rays of the sun. Its permanence takes place only until sunset. An Islamic-based psychological approach toward inner peace begins with redefining humans – their mission and their responsibility.

A human being is not summed up in the material realm and is not merely defined in physiological and neurological contexts with his or her attributes, including geographical, ethnic, racial, and physical characteristics. The realm of existence goes beyond what we have taken for granted in the material world. A human being is not merely a material being with no transcendental connection, and there is an immaterial component to human beings.

Everything in this world, ontologically speaking, is composed of two elements: the physical, which is directly perceptible and tangible through our senses, and the heavenly (*Malakoot*), which moves in line with the divine direction. A piece of stone, for instance, is characterized as an object, but it also possesses a heavenly dimension. Beyond *Malakoot* or the heavenly realm, there also lies a higher realm known as *Arsh* in Islamic terminology, which is not conceivable through our minds.

A spiritual Islamic psychological perspective on inner peace argues that human beings are defined by a journey (an elevating and transcendental journey) toward perfection and elevation, and in that pursuit would embrace *Marefat* (a term beyond knowledge and wisdom and intelligence with two characteristics: tranquility and imperturbability) – and the more they attain *Marefat*, the more they experience their true heavenly truth. (The truth is individuated in accordance with one's ontological and epistemological capacity but is ultimately linked to the Higher Truth.)

With more manifestation and crystallization of the heavenly truth, people get closer to God (not physically speaking) and experience *Qorb* (proximity toward God). *Qorb* is characterized through purification of the soul, where one mindfully, knowingly, and deliberately empties his or her heart from worldly attachments and belongings and attempts to enrich his or her soul by developing more connection to God. *Qorb* is also characterized through sincerity, authenticity, and genuineness in action, removing any signs of hypocrisy, pretentiousness, and ostentatiousness.

The more one's capacity for embracing the heavenly realm (*Malakoot*) grows, the more one acquires competencies toward psychological, spiritual, intellectual, and emotional empowerment. One's will becomes more empowered accordingly and finds a divine quiddity. In effect, many people may stand only in their own animalistic quiddity, and they may not go up to reach the elevated status of becoming a divine nature. The body becomes weak not in the literal sense of the word, but in the spiritual, because without *Qorb*, one cannot transcend the body's limitations.

Beyond the overarching theme of embracing *Malakoot*, Islam has other attributes and goals that lead toward well-being. One of these goals is to help people acquire a perspective that disallows them from misusing or abusing power. The world without power makes no sense, but the power conquered by egoism, egotism, arrogance, selfishness, hubris, utilitarianism, exploitation, and self-centeredness would bring havoc, destruction, annihilation, and despair. An Islam-based psychology elucidates the importance of self-management and self-regulation in giving direction to the use of power. One who feels needless and is saturated in hubris may set out to move in pursuit of power at any cost. One may feel powerful and yet in dire need of an obedience to the source of all powers, namely, God, and one may feel needless of an attachment to such a source. An Islamic-based psychological perspective on peace considers one of the main causes of arrogance and its destructive implications in one's feeling of needlessness. When one feels groundless and needless, one does not feel it necessary to abide by any laws and hence considers oneself entitled to do anything one wills.

Understanding one's need to be constantly and continuously connected to the authentic source of power (i.e., God) would help one observe the importance of self-management and self-regulation. Deep down, beneath human atrocities, human destructiveness, and human ferocities, there lies a relentless inattention toward the implications of selfishness, which takes place in an infatuation with one's feeling of needlessness and one's feeling of hubris in doing whatever one desires to do.

The spiritual journey is infinite, as it entails a journey toward God that has no end point. It constantly, incessantly, and continuously goes on. There is no single action where one can implement one's practical faith. Hazrat Zahra (Salamollah Alayha), in describing the available opportunities of spiritual growth in every single moment of life, indicates that true Muslims are characterized through their smiling faces, their kind and delicate hearts, and their compassion, kind words, and good deeds. The more one is in touch with one's spiritual performance and the more one is closely knitted to transcendental elevation, the more one becomes prepared for growth. One of the keys in putting this spiritual leap into effect is through doing and being good to others. Many Hadiths and several Quranic verses emphasize displaying kindness, graciousness, benevolence, munificence, and friendliness to others to the extent that Prophet Muhammad (*Sallalah alayhe va alehee va sallam*) considers one of the easiest and closest ways to God is the removal of sadness from the hearts of others.

In line with an attempt toward doing good to others, an Islamic perspective explicates the need for increasing awareness prior to every single decision. Human perfection, the Islamic perspective argues, does not lie in the progression of automatic, instinctual, and habitual ways of living but in the enhancement and enrichment of wise choices. One is mindfully responsible to monitor one's decisions, thoughts, feelings, and actions. In doing so, one is reminded of noticing the presence of God so that one is never alone.

Death, in an Islamic-based psychology, is not meant to be the end of life but the commencement of an eternal life. One becomes the total sum of one's choices. The more one's choices intermingle with awareness, virtue, piety, morality, and wisdom, the more one's path to perfection opens up.

An Islam-based psychology highlights the importance of simultaneously taking care of the soul and the body. Nourishment for the body transpires through the body-oriented means, whereas nourishment of the soul occurs through seeking connection to the source of all virtues and all of perfection, namely, God.

It is noteworthy that the conceptualization of heart and heartfulness unfolds an entirely new medium, language, and paradigm within the spiritual focus of Islamic psychology. Understanding the newness and uniqueness of this paradigm would provide significant implications from a psychological perspective.

Heart (*Qalb*) is not the physiological heart but the essence of human development facilitating the path toward salvation, emancipation, growth, and transcendence. There are at least 70 meanings and ramifications for

Qalb, including closed hearts, open hearts, locked hearts, contracted hearts, and expanded hearts. An important Quranic verse indicates that some people seemingly have hearts but are devoid of hearts:

> They have hearts with which they do not understand, they have eyes with which they do not see, and they have ears with which they do not hear. Those are like livestock; rather, they are more astray. It is they who are the heedless. (Al-A'raf, verse 179)

A Hadith from the leader of the faithful Imam Ali (Salavtollah Alayh) says, "People's hearts serve as capacities, the best of hearts are the ones with the most expansive capacities" (Hakimi, 1997, p. 69).

Heart constitutes the essence and the truth of humanness and serves as the most vitally existential base of human beings. Human guidance takes place through heart. The human soul can achieve its ascension through its divine heart and can go through descension by losing the divine heart.

Interestingly enough, a verse in the Holy Quran explicates that wakefulness and mindfulness in the Quranic sense belong to those who have hearts. The verse indicates that "[i]ndeed in that is a reminder for whoever has a heart or who listens while he is present in mind" (QAF, verse 37). In discussing the meaning of heart in the verse, Hakimi (2011, p. 296) quotes Majmaol Bahrein (Volume 2, p. 287), which says, "Heart in here is meant to be wisdom."

Hakimi then brings a Hadith from Imam Moosa Kazem (Salavatoollah Alayh) addressing Hesham, which says, "Oh Hesham, God says: in this there lies a reminder for the one who has heart namely that has wisdom and puts into practice his wisdom" (Tohafol Oqool, p. 287).

In continuation with exploring the nature of heart within the Islamic school of thought, Hakimi, Hakimi, and Hakimi (2011) also cite Allameh Majlesi and his exegesis on heart, which highlights the importance of revitalizing heart: "One must beautify the heart with divine practices of angels so heart can be empowered to obtain different degrees of perfection and achieve God's grace" (Beharol Anvar, Volume 70, pp. 33–36).

Hakimi et al. (2011) then present their elaborate study on multifaceted meanings of heart and offer strategies to enliven the heart based on Quranic verses and Hadiths. They enumerate at least seven ways to give rise to the heart's wakefulness and vivacity, including reflective silence; contemplation on one's actions and deeds; and reflection on existence, the cosmos, the stars, the sky, galaxies, mountains, birds, plants, and so forth.

In numerous Hadiths from Imam Ali (Salavatollah Alayh), the heart's liveliness is related to an exposure to spiritual reminders. Likewise, the thought of death would conquer the animalistic nature of Nafs and allow purification of the soul, and removal of hubris, greed, selfishness, arrogance, and jealousy and cultivation of modesty, compassion, spirituality, and wisdom would facilitate the process of heart's liveliness.

Correspondingly, another Hadith from Imam Sadegh (Alayhessalam) indicates the relationship between silence and one's prosperity, as silence, reflection, and contemplation would provide one with a phenomenological connection with heartfulness. Also, in Chapter Al-Hajj, verse 46, the Holy Quran delineates the essentiality of heart for understanding:

> Have they not traveled over the land so that they may have hearts by which they may apply reason or ears by which they may hear? Indeed it is not the eyes that turn blind but the hearts turn blind – those that are in the breasts!

An authentic, genuine, and sincere journey toward God without any pretentiousness, hypocrisy, and deception enhances one's capacity. This is the nature of life for humans and a central aspect of what is termed "mental" health. One of the essential keys in enhancing and revitalizing one's capacity lies in one's compassion toward the self and others. Again, a Hadith leader of the faithful Imam Ali (Salavtollah Alayh) indicates to "commit yourself with awareness and openness toward loving others, helping others, assisting others and solving their problems" (Hakimi, 1997, p. 70). In another Hadith from Prophet Muhammad (*Sallalaho alayhe va alehee va salaam*), the closest route to God is delineated through removing sadness from the other's heart, and this is done through compassion and mercy (Hakimi, 1997, p. 105).

Discussing the essence of compassion, peace, and mercy in an Islamic psychological perspective, Jafari (2006), an Iranian contemporary philosopher and scholar of Islam, cites Imam Ali with the following decrees on the rights of animals:

> Do not keep the animals and their children separate from one another.
> Make sure that you keep your nails short upon milking lest the animals may feel annoyed.
> If you happen to take the animals out for grazing, make sure that you walk them through the beautiful meadows if there are any.
>
> Rest assured that enough milk is left for the animal when milking.
> God will damn the one who uses profane language while addressing any animal.
> The governor can punish anyone who does not take care of his/her animal.
>
> (pp. 159–162)

Jafari (2006) then asks how a worldview that is so sensitive toward the rights of animals can be indifferent when dealing with human rights. He presents numerous examples from within the Islamic tradition to argue that Islam displays an essentially vital sensitivity toward the rights of any living creature, with the maximum possible rights for any human being.

In discussing the concept of heart (*Qalb*) within the Islamic spiritual psychological perspective, it is important to elucidate that the concept opens up an essentially different paradigm in comparison with other usages of heart in similar spiritual outlooks.

The premise of the conceptualization of heart (*Qalb*) in Islamic spirituality argues that there are two different entities for heart: one that belongs to the body and another that is affiliated with the soul. The former may be healthy and fine while the latter can be ill or vice versa. Take the case of a person of wisdom and mysticism with great virtues in action whose physical heart is ill while his heart (*Qalb*) of the soul is intact. The well-being of heart in the second sense requires awareness, mindfulness, purification, detachment, belonging, practice, and reliance.

Awareness goes back to cultivating the power of choices in relation to all kinds of decisions, behaviors, thoughts, and intentions. When people are at the mercy of their automatic, impulsive behaviors, they mainly come from a reactive position. Mindfulness supports and consolidates the awareness as it helps one's choices to be connected to the splendor of the. Purification consists in a deliberate attempt to cleanse one's heart from anything that blocks or stops the spiritual development. Jealousy, hubris, greed, arrogance, selfishness, egoism, and oppression are some of the examples that impede the process of achieving a peace-oriented heart. Consequently, one needs to constantly be mindful of what he or she does and says to ensure that the termites of heartlessness do not nest in his or her soul. Purification also requires a self-regulated and self-disciplined program where one can constantly monitor his or her actions, thoughts, and behaviors. This should not be confused with an obsession where someone is constantly bombarded by distressing thoughts and behaviors.

Purification takes place deliberately, freely, and mindfully. Imam Alia has beautifully explicated that "detachment is not that you should not own anything, detachment is that nothing should own you." A healthy heart needs to be able to consciously and mindfully be prepared to detach all forms of belongings, wishes, thoughts, desires, and so on to make sure that he or she is managed by them.

When the heart is overcome by debilitating forces of helplessness, despair, excessiveness, extremism, lavishness, and arrogance, the heart loses its liveliness and vivacity and gets embroiled in the dark chambers of destructive engagements. Practicing detachment would elevate one's heart's receptiveness in a journey toward self-empowerment, self-enrichment, and self-revitalization.

In an Islamic context, mindfulness unfolds its power in a lively phenomenological connection to the presence of God. God is closer to one than anything else. The Holy Quran states, "It was We Who created man, and We know what dark suggestions his soul makes to him: for We are nearer to him than (his) jugular vein. We are nearer to him than (his) jugular vein." (Surah Qaf, the Letter, 50, verse 16).

Reliance refers to trust in God in all circumstances and understanding that God will be the best supporter, the best listener, and the best viewer. Rumi delineates the relationship in the following ways:

> Each moment contains
> a hundred messages from God:
> To every cry of "Oh Lord,"
> He answers a hundred times, "I am here." (Rumi, I, p. 1578)

Taking care of the soul stands at the forefront of a leading spiritual life. Prophet Mohammad (*Sallal alayhe va alehee va salaam*) indicates that "[t]here is a polish for everything, and the polish for the heart is the remembrance of God." Remembrance of God, from a spiritual and mystical perspective, can serve as a panacea to bring calmness, tranquility, and peace to one's heart. Hearts can be locked and shut down when they do not receive spiritual liveliness and exhilaration. When one's heart is clouded and shrouded by egoism and obsession with the likes and belongings of the transient world, one's vision will be taken over by impulses, emotional hastiness, emotional abduction, and mindless forms of reactivity. The more one's heart is steeped in the materialistic inclinations, the more one's heart's capacity experiences a regression toward carnal desires, animalistic tendencies, and egotistic propensities.

Imam Ali (*Salavatollah alayh*), the leader of the faithful, in a letter to his son Imam Hassan Mojtab (*Alahyessalam*) invites him to enliven his heart through being receptive to illuminating pearls of spirituality, wisdom, and transcendental advice.

Rumi calls for removing anxiety, worries, and obsessions and says, "Let go of your worries and be completely clear-hearted, like the face of a mirror that contains no images. When it is empty of forms, all forms are contained within it. No face would be ashamed to be so clear."

Inner peace in an Islamic spiritual context is placed in the education of a healthy heart. The Holy Quran lays emphasis on understanding the functions of heart (*Qalb*), educating the heart, and modifying and revising the heart.

Almost 50 types of heart have been presented in the Holy Quran. Elaborating on these different types of hearts, Hakimi, Hakimi, and Hakimi (2007) indicate that each of the verses with a thematic analysis on heart explicates the elements that contribute to the formation of any of these hearts.

An Islamic psychological perspective on peace articulates that global peace requires an in-depth move toward the human heart's purification and liveliness. The heart's liveliness lies in conscious and coherent attempts to purify, enhance, and enrich one's heart. This, ipso facto, necessitates a leap beyond the pretentious self being mired with fear, anxiety, selfishness, hubris, and arrogance.

When one is stuck in the falsehood of selfishness, one cannot be separated from the narrowness of one's mindset and fails to join the liberating movement of inner peace. A continuous obsession with fears and anxiety along with a stretched-out focus on materialism would lead to self- imprisonment. One may speak of peace and yet be embroiled and encumbered with the burden of inner conflicts and inner tension.

The Holy Quran refers to a healthy heart. Chapter Al-Saffat, verse 84, describes Abraham's heart when it says, "he came to his Lord with a sound heart.".

A sound and healthy heart is a heart devoid of animalistic tendencies, with a remembrance of God.

Parallel with the discussion on creating a sound and healthy heart, one can expand one's level of Qalb's elevation through strategies such as Dhikr. Dhikr explicates an ongoing connectedness and remembrance of God. Salavat and Dhikr may open up Qalb and make it ready to experience the spiritual illumination. Dhikr can also be classified in several layers; one is the language-oriented Dhikr followed by the Qalb-oriented Dhikr.

There has been a misrepresentation of Islam's message in current culture that merits reconciling. In his book *The Clash of Civilizations and the Remaking of the World Order* (1996, p. 258), Huntington discusses "Islamic civilization" and indicates that "Muslim bellicosity and violence are late twentieth-century facts which neither Muslims nor non-Muslims can deny." In discussing the comments and allegations, including those by Huntington, Spariosu (2004, p. 51) writes,

The traditional greeting among Muslims is "Peace be with you" (Al-Salam Alei-kum) or that Sufi teachings do not condone violence and conflict any more than their Buddhist, Taoist, or Christian counterparts do. For example, the prophet Muhammad says: "If a man gives up quarreling when he is in the wrong, a house will be built for him in Paradise. But if a man gives up a conflict even when he is in the right, a house will be built for him in the loftiest of Paradise" (Frager & Fadiman, 1997, p. 84).

If anything, Huntington's arguments highlight the ignorance of even well-trained Westerners about other cultures and religions (not to mention their own) and the urgent need for educating the world's youth about each other's – and their own – cultural traditions (p. 51).

In line with an awareness of making a distinction between misrepresentation of spirituality and the nature of spirituality, Vaillant (2008) writes,

> The ongoing bloody conflict between the Sunni Muslims and the Shiite Muslims over control of Iraq cannot be blamed on the unifying spiritual vision of the Qur'an. When faith is about selfish politics, or when projection replaces empathy, it becomes destructive. As with paranoia, selfishness is not susceptible to another's point of view. Faith, then, is not the danger; the danger is the lack of empathy and the false beliefs of those who profess faith. Inner illumination, to be safe, must perceive others accurately. (p. 81)

Elaborating on the necessity of making a distinction between the misrepresentations of spirituality and religiosity that take place in the name of religions and spirituality and the pristine substance of spirituality and religiosity, Vaillant (2008) articulates,

> In sum, whenever the quest for loving inner illumination becomes a fanatical "all about me" belief system, the result is catastrophe. The intolerant faith of the "moral majority" in the contemporary United States, of the Taliban in Afghanistan, of the murderous Jewish Law in the Book of Deuteronomy, and of the Catholic Inquisition is more typical of a selfish quest for power than of the billions of ordinary people who "do" religious faith and trust a loving universe. (p. 81)

Understanding the vital role of heartfulness in developing an orientation toward compassion, empathy, kindness, love, and peace is repeatedly cited and displayed in the Islamic perspective on peace. Heartfulness would provide one with a deep interest and serious attempt to revise one's position in the world to ensure that one's performance is enhanced daily in terms of heart-oriented criteria, not the materialist yardsticks. This requires a mindful engagement in offering munificence and benevolence to everyone in the world, so much so that the Prophet of Islam Hazrat Mohammad (*Salavtollah alayhe va alehee ajmaeen*) considers the removal of sadness from the other's hearts as one of the closest paths to achieving God's satisfaction. To break one's heart, to insult others, to depreciate other people, and to display condescending behavior are among the seriously noxious elements that impede the process of the heart's liveliness.

Heartfulness is described as the substance of one's enhancement toward growth, perfection, transcendence, and betterment. The realm of heart is an infinitely open domain that has no halting point. It can continuously grow through actions, thoughts, emotions, behaviors, and even intentionality. Positive intentionality with an orientation toward doing good unto others can expand one's heart, as other signs of munificence and compassion can substantiate the vivacity of one's heartfulness.

Epilogue

Peace requires a recondite understanding of humanness and its innerness. When taken superficially, one may come up with strategies and remedies that might espouse controlling, regulating, and modulating human interaction for a short period of time at the cost of ignoring the clandestinely profound forces within the human psyche.

A rigorous understanding of peace may help us go back to our togetherness and our common roots and may allow us to hear the tintinnabulation of the deeply shaped nuance of our communality. This may be the sine qua non of exploring the innate subtlety and beauty of our heartfulness. The deluge of mind-induced operations and their consequential ramifications may have brought us to a mindless state of forgetting about the vitality of heart.

Our enterprises and our tasks may have entrenched us in an abyss of nearsightedness where our concerns and propensities have mainly coiled around mind-derived paraphernalia.

Our forgetfulness and our mindlessness have combined mindsets and parameters that have hampered the process of our search in the infinite human possibilities within the human soul and its infinitely alive realm of activities. Our modes of livingness and our modalities of connectedness have, therefore, mainly been confined to linear, competitive, speculative, analytical, and mind-oriented operations within the realm of the visible.

Our gradual exposure to the mentality of linearity and causality may have imposed a soporific negligence that would be silently or clamorously awakened at the mercy of tragic events such as tornadoes, terrorism, genocide, and a worldwide pandemic. Our phenomenological encounter with the immediacy and inevitability of death and mortality may bring a ripple of a dormant gaze at the essentiality of addressing our existential angst, our ontological meaning, and our meaningfulness or meaninglessness.

An erudite examination of peace can help us travel through the mostly unfrequented lands of innerness where beauty, awe, glory, and the elevation of the soul loom at the apex of liveliness.

Heartfulness provides us with the deepest ever quest of humanness in the infinite world of the spirit. Our habituation in the circle of materialism has distanced us from an open journey within the innerness where peace and heartfulness celebrate their synergy in giving rise to human personality's coherence, wholeness, wellness, well-being, and health.

Our yearning for heartfulness may not have been heard by the domineering materialistic discourses of power, hegemony, consumerism, greed, hubris, arrogance, discrimination, injustice, oppression, and coercion but have sporadically and cogently appeared in our works of art, literature, poetry, films, and music, as well as our aesthetic cravings.

Heartfulness may help us revisit our postulated strategies for our creation, our decisions, and our policies.

For a global peace to happen, heartfulness can serve as a panacea, as a key to unlock the shutdown doors of our emotional, our intellectual, and our spiritual togetherness.

Heartfulness may facilitate the process of emotional maturity and leading intellectual maturity toward achieving spiritual maturity.

Heartfulness can substantiate the reason for our commonly felt ties, for our shared values and shared beliefs.

World peace may unfold its sustainable possibility in light of mindful attempts to bring heartfulness into our existential estrangement.

Bibliography

Abbass, A. (2002). Intensive short-term dynamic psychotherapy in a private psychiatric office: Clinical and cost effectiveness. *American Journal of Psychotherapy*, 56, 225–232.

(2003). The cost-effectiveness of short-term dynamic psychotherapy. *Journal of Pharmacoeconomics and Outcomes Research*, 3, 535–539.

Abbass, A., Campbell, S., Magee, K., Lenzer, I., Hann, G., & Tarzwell, R. (2010). Cost savings of treatment of medically unexplained symptoms using intensive short-term dynamic psychotherapy (ISTDP) by a hospital emergency department. *Archives of Medical Psychology*, 2, 34–44.

Abbass, A., Kisely, S., & Kroenke, K. (2009). Short-term psychodynamic psychotherapy for somatic symptom disorders: A systematic review and meta-analysis. *Psychotherapy and Psychosomatics*, 78, 265–274.

Abbass, A., Lovas, D., & Purdy, A. (2008). Direct diagnosis and management of emotional factors in the chronic headache patient. *Cephalalgia*, 28, 1305–1314.

Abu-Rabi, I. M. (1996). *Intellectual origins of Islamic resurgence in the modern Arab world*. Albany, NY: State University of New York at Albany.

Ainsworth, M. D. S. (1982). Attachment: Retrospect and prospect. In C. M. Parkes & J. Stevenson-Hinde (Eds.), *The place of attachment in human behavior* (pp. 3–30). New York: Basic Books.

Albee, G. W. (1981). Politics, power, prevention, and social change. In J. M. Joffee & G. W. Albee (Eds.), *Prevention through political action and social change* (pp. 5–25). Hanover, NH: University Press of New England.

Allport, G. W. (1955). *Becoming: Basic considerations for a psychology of personality*. New Haven, CT: Yale University Press.

American Psychiatric Association. (2000). *Diagnostic and statistical manual of mental disorders DSM-IV-TR* (4th ed., text revision). Washington, DC: American Psychiatric Association.

Amir, M., Kaplan, Z., Neumann, L., Sharabani, R., Shani, N., & Buskila, D. (1997). Posttraumatic stress disorder, tenderness and fibromyalgia. *Journal of Psychosomatic Research*, 42, 607–613.

Anda, R. F., Felitti, V. J., Bremner, J. D., Walker, J. D., Whitfield, C., Perry, B. D., ... Giles, W. H. (2006). The enduring effects of abuse and related adverse experiences in childhood: A convergence of evidence from

96 *Bibliography*

neurobiology and epidemiology. *European Archives of Psychiatry and Clinical Neuroscience*, 256, 174–186.

Anderson, C. A., & Bushman, B. J. (1997). External validity of "trivial" experiments: The case of laboratory aggression. *Review of General Psychology*, 1, 19–41.

(2002). Media violence and societal violence. *Science*, 295, 2377–2378.

Anderson, C. A., Shibuya, A., Ihori, N., Swing, E. L., Bushman, B. J., Sakamoto, A., . . . Saleem, M. (2010). Violent video-game effects on aggression, empathy, and prosocial behavior in Eastern and Western countries. *Psychological Bulletin*, 136, 151–173.

Archer, J. (2000). Sex differences in aggression between heterosexual partners: A meta-analytic review. *Psychological Bulletin*, 126, 651–680.

Armstrong, D. M. (1968). *A materialist theory of the mind*. London: Routledge & Kegan Paul.

Armstrong, K. (2003). *The spiral staircase: My climb out of darkness*. New York: Knopf.

Austin, E. J., & Deary, I. J. (2002). Personality dispositions. In R. J. Sternberg (Ed.), *Why smart people can be so stupid* (pp. 187–211). New Haven, CT: Yale University Press.

Avicenna. (1404 Hejri). *Taaleeqaat*. Abdolrahman Badavee.

Azar, B. (2001). A new take on psychoneuroimmunology. *Monitor on Psychology*, 32(11), 34–36.

Babeveyh, M. I. (1983). *Maaneeol Akhbar*. Qom, Iran: Jamee Modareseene Hoze Elmiyeh Qom.

(2007). *Elalalo ssharaeh*. Qom, Iran: Davari.

Baer, R. A. (2007). Mindfulness, assessment, and transdiagnostic processes. *Psychological Inquiry*, 18, 238–242.

Baliki, M. N., Petre, B., Torbey, S., Herrmann, K. M., Huang, L., Schnitzer, T. J., . . . Apkarian, V. (2012). Corticostriatal functional connectivity predicts transition to chronic back pain. *Nature Neuroscience*, 15, 1117–1119.

Ballantyne, J. C., Fishman, S. M., & Abdi, S. (2002). *The Massachusetts General Hospital handbook of pain management* (2nd ed.). New York: Lippincott Williams & Wilkins.

Bandura, A. (1977a). Self-efficacy: Toward a unifying theory of behavioral change. *Psychological Review*, 84, 191–215.

(1977b). *Social learning theory*. Englewood Cliffs, NJ: Prentice Hall.

Banister, P., Burman, E., Parker, I., Taylor. M., & Tindall, C. (1994). *Qualitative methods in psychology: A research guide*. Buckingham, UK: Open University Press.

Baron, R. A. (1976). The reduction of human aggression: A field study of the influence of incompatible reactions. *Journal of Applied Social Psychology*, 6, 260–74.

Baron, R. A., & Richardson, D. R. (1994). *Human aggression* (2nd ed.). New York: Plenum Press.

Beauregard, M., & O'Leary, D. (2007). *The spiritual brain: A neuroscientist's case for the existence of the soul*. New York: HarperOne.

Beckham, J. C., Crawford, A. L., Feldman, M. E., Kirby, A. C., Hertzberg, M. A., Davidson, J. R., & Moore, S. D. (1997). Chronic posttraumatic stress disorder and chronic pain in Vietnam combat veterans. *Journal of Psychosomatic Research*, 43, 379–389.

Benson, H., Beary, J. F., & Carol, M. P. (1974). The relaxation response. *Psychiatry*, 37, 37–46.

Berkowitz, L. (1989). Frustration-aggression hypothesis: Examination and reformulation. *Psychological Bulletin*, 106, 59–73.

Berkowitz, L., & LePage, A. (1967). Weapons as aggression-eliciting stimuli. *Journal of Personality and Social Psychology*, 7, 202–207.

Bernal, J. D. (1954). *Science in history*. New York: Hawthorn Books.

Bettencourt, B. A., & Miller, N. (1996). Gender differences in aggression as a function of provocation: A meta-analysis. *Psychological Bulletin*, 119, 422–447.

Boos, N., Semmer, N., Elfering, A., Schade, V., Gal, I., Zanetti, M., . . . Main, C. J. (2000). Natural history of individuals with asymptomatic disc abnormalities in magnetic resonance imaging: Predictors of low back pain–related medical consultation and work incapacity. *Spine*, 25, 1484–1492.

Borenstein, D. G., O'Mara, J. W., Jr., Boden, S. D., Lauerman, W. C., Jacobson, A., Platenberg, C., . . . Wiesel, S. W. (2001). The value of magnetic resonance imaging of the lumbar spine to predict low-back pain in asymptomatic subjects: A seven-year follow-up study. *Journal of Bone and Joint Surgery* (American), 83-A, 1306–1311.

Bowlby, J. (1954). *Maternal care and mental health*. Washington, DC: World Health Organization.

(1973). Separation: *Anxiety and anger*. New York: Basic Books.

Brewer, J., Bowen, S., Smith, J., Marlatt, G., & Potenza, M. (2010). Response to Commentaries. *Addiction*, 105, 1709–1710.

Brewer, J. A., Worhunsky, P. D., Gray, J. R., Tang, Y., Weber, J., & Kober, H. (2011). Meditation experience is associated with differences in default mode network activity and connectivity. *Proceedings of the National Academy of Sciences*, 108, 20254–20259.

Buhner, S. H. (2004). *The secret teachings of plants: The intelligence of the heart in the direct perception of nature*. Rochester, VT: Bear and Company.

Burger, A. J., Schubiner, H., Carty, J., Valentino, D., Sklar, E., Hyde-Nolan, M., . . . Lumley, M. A. (2011, March). Outcomes and predictors of a novel emotional awareness and expression treatment for chronic pain. Paper presented at the Annual Meeting of the American Psychosomatic Society, San Antonio, TX.

Bushman, B. J. (1997). Effects of alcohol on human aggression: Validity of proposed explanations. In D. Fuller, R. Dietrich, & E. Gottheil (Eds.), *Recent developments in alcoholism: Alcohol and violence* (Vol. 13, pp. 227–243). New York: Plenum Press.

Bushman, B. J., & Baumeister, R. F. (1998). Threatened egotism, narcissism, self-esteem, and direct and displaced aggression: Does self-love or self-hate lead to violence? *Journal of Personality and Social Psychology*, 75, 219–229.

Bushman, B. J., Baumeister, R. F., Thomaes, S., Ryu, E., Begeer, S., & West, S. G. (2009). Looking again, and harder, for a link between low self-esteem and aggression. *Journal of Personality*, 77, 427–446.

Bushman, B. J., & Huesmann, L. R. (2010). Aggression. In S. T. Fiske, D. T. Gilbert, & G. Lindzey (Eds.), *Handbook of social psychology* (5th ed., pp. 833–863). New York: John Wiley & Sons.

Bruner, J. (1986). *Actual minds, possible worlds*. Cambridge, MA: Harvard University Press.

Burger, J. M. (1992). *Desire for control: Personality, social, and clinical perspectives*. New York: Plenum Press.

Burns, J. W., Quartana, P., Gilliam, W., Gray, E., Matsuura, J., Nappi, C., … Lofland, K. (2008). Effects of anger suppression on pain severity and pain behaviors among chronic pain patients: Evaluation of an ironic process model. *Health Psychology*, 27, 645–652.

Buss, A. H., & Perry, M. (1992). The Aggression Questionnaire. *Journal of Personality and Social Psychology*, 63, 452–459.

Campbell, J. (1949/2008). *The hero with a thousand faces*. Princeton, NJ: Princeton University Press.

Caplan, G. (1974). *Support systems and community mental health: Lectures on concept development*. New York: Behavioral Publications.

Carlson, M., Marcus-Newhall, A., & Miller, N. (1990). Effects of situational aggression cues: A quantitative review. *Journal of Personality and Social Psychology*, 58, 622–633.

Carnagey, N. L., & Anderson, C. A. (2005). The effects of reward and punishment in violent video games on aggressive affect, cognition, and behavior. *Psychological Science*, 16, 882–889.

Carpendale, J., & Krebs, D. L. (1995). Variations in the level of moral judgment as a function of type of dilemma and moral choice. *Journal of Personality*, 63, 289–313.

Carrington, D. (2020). Coronavirus: "Nature is sending us a message," says UN environmental chief. *The Guardian*, March 25. www.theguardian.com/world/2020/mar/25/coronavirus-nature-is-sending-us-a-message-says-un-environment-chief

Cassel, J. (1976). The contribution of the social environment to host resistance: The fourth Wade Hampton Frost lecture. *American Journal of Epidemiology*, 104, 107–123.

Center on the Developing Child, Harvard University. (2020). Neglect. https://developingchild.harvard.edu/science/deep-dives/neglect/

Cherkin, D. C., Eisenberg, D., Sherman, K. J., Barlow, W., Kaptchuk, T. J., Street, J., & Deyo, R. A. (2001). Randomized trial comparing traditional Chinese medical acupuncture, therapeutic massage, and self-care education for chronic low back pain. *Archives of Internal Medicine*, 161, 1081–1088.

Christie, D. J., Tint, B. S., Wagner, R. V., & Winter, D. D. (2008). Peace psychology for a peaceful world. *American Psychologist*, 63, 540–552.

Churchland, P. (1987). *Matter and consciousness: An introduction to the philosophy of mind*. Cambridge, MA: MIT Press.

Cobb, S. (1976). Social support as a moderator of life stress. *Psychosomatic Medicine*, 38, 300–313.

Collins, S. (1982). *Selfless persons*. Cambridge: Cambridge University Press.

Collins, R. L., Quigley, B., & Leonard, K. (2007). Women's physical aggression in bars: An event-based examination of precipitants and predictors of severity. *Aggressive Behavior*, 33, 304–313.

Cottinghan, J. (2020). What is the soul if not a better version of ourselves? *Aeon*. https://bit.ly/39nsrBP

Coughlin Della Selva, P. (1996). *Intensive short-term dynamic psychotherapy: Theory and practice*. New York: John Wiley & Sons.

Coughlin Della Selva, P., & Malan, D. (2006). *Lives transformed: A revolutionary method of dynamic psychotherapy*. London: Karnac Books.

Creel, H. G. (1960). *Confucius and the Chinese way*. New York: Harper Torchbooks.

Crick, N. R., & Grotpeter, J. K. (1995). Relational aggression, gender, and social-psychological adjustment. *Child Development*, 66, 710–722.

Crockett, M., Kappes, A., & Nussberger, A.-M. (2018). Pandemics and the psychology of uncertainty. World Economic Forum. www.weforum.org/agenda/2018/08/the- psychology-of-pandemics

Crum, A., & Lyddy, C. (2014). De-stressing stress: The power of mindsets and the art of stressing mindfully. In A. N. Ie, C. T. Ngnoumen, & E. J. Langer (Eds.), *The handbook of mindfulness* (pp. 948–963). Hoboken, NJ: John Wiley & Sons.

Csikszentmihalyi, M. (1990). *Flow: The psychology of optimal experience*. New York: HarperCollins.

Cushman, P. (1990). Why the self is empty: Toward a historically situated psychology. *American Psychologist*, 45, 599–611.

Dahl, J., & Lundgren, T. (2006). *Living beyond your pain: Using acceptance and commitment therapy to ease chronic pain*. Oakland, CA: New Harbinger.

Dale, G. A., & Wrisberg, C. A. (1996). The use of a performance profiling technique in a team setting: Getting athletes and coaches on the "same page." *The Sport Psychologist*, 10, 261–277.

Damasio, A. (1994). *Descartes' error: Emotion, reason, and the human brain*. New York: Putnam.

(2003). *Looking for Spinoza: Joy, sorrow, and the feeling brain*. New York: Houghton Mifflin Harcourt.

Danziger, K. (1990). *Constructing the subject: Historical origins of psychological research*. Cambridge: Cambridge University Press.

Davanloo, H. (1978). *Basic principles and techniques in short-term dynamic psychotherapy*. New York: Spectrum Press.

(1990). *Unlocking the unconscious*. New York, NY: Wiley Press.

(1999). Intensive short-term dynamic psychotherapy—central dynamic sequences. *International Journal of Intensive Short-Term Dynamic Psychotherapy*, 13, 211–262.

De Jachger, H., Di Paolo, E., & Gallagher, S. (2010). Can social interaction constitute social cognition? *Trends in Cognitive Sciences*, 14, 441–447.

Derbyshire, S. W. G., Whalley, M. G., Stenger, V. A., & Oakley, D. A. (2004). Cerebral activation during hypnotically induced and imagined pain. *Neuroimage*, 23, 392–401.

Derrida, J. (1976). *Of grammatology*. Baltimore, MD: Johns Hopkins University Press.

de Saint-Exupéry, A. (1943). *The little prince*. New York: Harcourt, Brace and World.

Deyo, R. A., Mirza, S. K., Turner, J. A., & Martin, B. I. (2009). Overtreating chronic back pain: Time to back off? *Journal of the American Board of Family Medicine*, 22, 62–68.

DiBerardinis, J. D., Barwind, J., Flanninam, R. R., & Jenkins, V. (1983). Enhanced interpersonal relation as predictor of athletic performance. *International Journal of Sport Psychology*, 14, 243–51.

Dill, K. E., Anderson, C. A., Anderson, K. B., & Deuser, W. E. (1997). Effects of aggressive personality on social expectations and social perceptions. *Journal of Research in Personality*, 31, 272–292.

Ditto, B., Eclache, M., & Goldman, N. (2006). Short-term autonomic and cardiovascular effects of mindfulness body scan meditation. *Annals of Behavioral Medicine*, 32, 227–234.

Dobkin, P. L. (2008). Mindfulness-based stress reduction: What processes are at work? *Complementary Therapies in Clinical Practice*, 14, 8–16.

Dodge, K. A. (1980). Social cognition and children's aggressive behavior. *Child Development*, 51, 620–635.

Dollard, J., & Miller, N. (1950). *Personality and psychotherapy: An analysis in terms of learning, thinking, and culture*. New York: McGraw-Hill.

Dollard, J., Doob, L., Miller, N., Mowrer, O., & Sears, R. (1939). *Frustration and aggression*. New Haven, CT: Yale University Press.

Du Bois, W. D., & Wright, R. D. (2002). What is humanistic sociology? *The American Sociologist*, 33(4), 5–36.

Durkheim, E. (1951). *Suicide: A study in sociology*. Trans. J. A. Spaulding & G. Simpson. New York: Free Press. (Original work published 1897)

Ebert, M. H., & Kerns, R. D. (Eds.). (2011). *Behavioral and psychopharmacologic pain management*. Cambridge: Cambridge University Press.

Eccleston, C., de C. Williams, A. C., & Morley, S. (2009). Psychological therapies for the management of chronic pain (excluding headache) in adults. *Cochrane Database of Systematic Reviews*, art. no. CD007407. doi:10.1002/14651858.CD007407.pub2

Ehrenreich, B. (2009). *Bright-sided: How the relentless promotion of positive thinking has undermined America*. New York: Metropolitan Books.

Eisenberger, N. I., Jarcho, J. M., Lieberman, M. D., & Naliboff, B. D. (2006). An experimental study of shared sensitivity to physical pain and social rejection. *PAIN*, 126, 132–138.

Eisenberger, N. I., Lieberman, M. D., & Williams, K. D. (2003). Does rejection hurt? An fMRI study of social exclusion. *Science*, 302, 290–292.

Epstein, S. (1998). *Constructive thinking: The key to emotional intelligence.* Westport, CT: Praeger.

Etheredge, L. S. (2005). Wisdom in public policy. In R. Sternberg & J. Jordan (Eds.), *Handbook of mindfulness* (pp. 297–329). New York: Cambridge University Press.

Fatemi, S. M. (2014). Exemplifying a shift of paradigm: Exploring the psychology of possibility and embracing the instability of knowing. In A. Ie, C. T. Ngoumen, & E. J. Langer (Eds.), *The handbook of mindfulness* (pp. 115–138). Hoboken, NJ: Wiley.

(Ed.). (2016). *Critical mindfulness: Exploring Langerian models.* New York: Springer.

(2018). Integrating Duaa Arafaa and other Shia teachings into psychotherapy. In C. York Al-Karam (Ed.), *Islamically integrated psychotherapy: Uniting faith and professional practice* (pp. 275–291). West Conshohocken, PA: Templeton Press.

Fineburg, A. (2004). Introducing positive psychology to the introductory psychology student. In P. A. Linley & S. Joseph (Eds.), *Positive psychology in practice.* Hoboken, NJ: John Wiley & Sons.

Finger, S. (1994). *Origins of neuroscience: A history of explorations into brain function.* Oxford: Oxford University Press.

Fischer, C. T. (2006). *Qualitative research methods for psychologists: Introduction through empirical studies.* San Diego, CA: Academic Press.

Frankl, V. E. (1963). *Man's search for meaning: An introduction to logotherapy.* New York: Washington Square.

(1967). Logotherapy and existentialism. *Psychotherapy: Theory, Research & Practice,* 4, 138–142.

Freud, S. (1930). *Civilization and its discontents.* New York: Norton.

(1918). Letter from Sigmund Freud to Oskar Pfister, October 9, 1918. *The International Psycho-Analytical Library,* 59, 61–63.

(1927). *The future of an illusion.* London: Hogarth Press.

(1932). Letter to Albert Einstein, September 1932. (Reprinted in *Great political thinkers: Plato to the present,* pp. 804–810, by W. Ebenstein, Ed., 1951, New York: Rinehart)

(1950). *Beyond the pleasure principle.* New York: Liveright.

(1962). *Civilization and its discontents.* New York: Norton.

(1999). *The standard edition of the complete psychological works of Sigmund Freud* (24 vols.). Ed. J. Strachey. New York: Vintage.

Gadamer, H. (1988). *Truth and method.* New York: Crossroad. (Original work published 1965, 1975; English)

Gailliot, M. T., & Baumeister, R. F. (2007). The physiology of willpower: Linking blood glucose to self-control. *Personality and Social Psychology Review,* 11, 303–327).

Garland, E. L. (2013). *Mindfulness-oriented recovery enhancement for addiction, stress, and pain.* Washington, DC: NASW Press.

Gardner, M. (1993). *The healing revelations of Mary Baker Eddy.* Amherst, NY: Prometheus Books.

Geen, R. G., & Quanty, M. B. (1977). The catharsis of aggression: An evaluation of a hypothesis. In L. Berkowitz (Ed.), *Advances in experimental social psychology* (Vol. 10, pp. 1–37). New York: Academic Press.

Gergen, K. J. (1990). Towards a postmodern psychology. *Humanistic Psychologist*, 18, 23–34.

Giancola, P. R. (2000). Executive functioning: A conceptual framework for alcohol-related aggression. *Experimental Clinical Psychopharmacology*, 8, 576–597.

Gilbert, D. T. (1991). How mental systems believe. *American Psychologist*, 46, 107–119.

Gillis, M. E., Lumley, M. A., Mosley-Williams, A., Leisen, J. C. C., & Roehrs, T. (2006). The health effects of at-home written emotional disclosure in fibromyalgia: A randomized trial. *Annals of Behavioral Medicine*, 32(2), 135–146.

Ginges, J., Atran, S., Sachdeva, A., & Medin, D. (2011). Psychology out of the laboratory: The challenge of violent extremism. *American Psychologist*, 66, 507–519.

Glaser, R., & Kiecolt-Glaser, J. K. (1994). *Handbook of human stress and immunity*. New York: Academic Press.

Glass, D. C., and Singer, J. E. (1972). *Urban stress: Experiments on noise and social stressors*. New York: Academic Press.

Goldenberg, D. L., Burckhardt, C., & Crofford, L. (2004). Management of fibromyalgia syndrome. *Journal of the American Medical Association*, 292, 2388–2395.

Goldfried, M. R., & Davison, G. S. (1976). *Clinical behavior therapy*. New York: Holt, Rinehart & Winston.

Goldman, R. H., Stason, W. B., Park, S. K., Kim, R., Schnyer, R. N., Davis, R. B., . . . Kaptchuk, T. J. (2008). Acupuncture for treatment of persistent arm pain due to repetitive use: A randomized controlled clinical trial. *Clinical Journal of Pain*, 24, 211–218.

Goldstein, J. (1993). *Insight meditation: A psychology of freedom*. Boston: Shambhala.

Gracely, R. H., Petzke, F., Wolf, J. M., & Clauw, D. J. (2002). Functional magnetic resonance imaging evidence of augmented pain processing in fibromyalgia. *Arthritis and Rheumatism*, 46, 1333–1343.

Gray, C. (2007). *War, peace and international relations: An introduction to strategic history*. New York: Routlege.

Grigorenko, E. L., & Lockery, D. (2002). Smart is as stupid does: Exploring bases of erroneous reasoning of smart people regarding learning and other disabilities. In R. J. Sternberg (Ed.), *Why smart people can be so stupid* (pp. 159–186). New Haven, CT: Yale University Press.

Grossman, P., Tiefenthaler-Gilmer, U., Raysz, A., & Kesper, U. (2007). Mindfulness training as an intervention for fibromyalgia: Evidence of post-intervention and 3-year follow-up benefits in well-being. *Psychotherapy and Psychosomatics*, 76, 226–233.

Guarneri, M. (2006). *The heart speaks: A cardiologist reveals the secret language of healing.* New York: Touchstone.

Habermas, J. (1972). *Knowledge and human interests.* Trans. J. J. Shapiro. Boston: Beacon Press. (Original work published 1968)

(1973). *Legitimation crisis.* Boston: Beacon Press.

(1975). *Legitimation crisis.* Boston: Beacon Press. (Original work published 1973)

Hadler, N. M. (2009). *Stabbed in the back: Confronting back pain in an overtreated society.* Raleigh: University of North Carolina Press.

Ha'iri Yazdi, M. (1992). *The principles of epistemology in Islamic philosophy.* Albany: State University of New York Press.

Hakimi, M. R. (1997). *Ejtehad Va Taghleed dar falsafe (Ejtehad or imitation in philosophy).* Qom, Iran: Daeele Ma.

(2004). *Elaheeyate Elahee va elaheeyate basharee (Islamic theology and man driven theology).* Qom, Iran: Daleele Ma.

(2013). *Ejtehad va taqleed dar falsafe (Ijtihad and mimicry in philosophy).* Qom, Iran: Daleele Ma.

Hakimi, M. R., Hakimi, A., & Hakimi, M. (2005). *Alhayat (Life).* Qom, Iran: Daleele Ma.

(2007). *Alhayat (Life).* Qom, Iran: Daleele Ma.

(2011). *Alhayat (Life).* Qom, Iran: Daleele Ma.

Hall, T. (1998). *Seeking a focus on joy in the field of psychology. New York Times,* April 28, section F, p. 7.

Hanh, T. N. (1976). *The miracle of mindfulness: A manual for meditation.* Boston: Beacon Press.

Harlow, H. F., Dodsworth, R. O., & Harlow, M. K. (1965). Total social isolation in monkeys. *Proceedings of the National Academy of Sciences of the United States of America.* www.ncbi.nlm.nih.gov/pmc/articles/PMC285801/pdf/pnas00159-0105.pdf

Harrani, H. E. S. (1984). *TohafolOqool anAle Rasool (Salavatollahalayh).* Beruit, Lebanon: Darol Eyha Atorath Alarabi.

Harre, R., & Secord, P. F. (1972). *The explanation of social behavior.* Oxford: Basil Blackwell.

Harvey, J. H., and Weary, G. (1984). Current issues in attribution theory and research. *Annual Review of Psychology,* 35, 427–459.

Heidegger, M. (1959). *An introduction to metaphysics.* New Haven, CT: Yale University Press.

(1995). *The fundamental concepts of metaphysics: World, finitude, solitude.* Bloomington: Indiana University Press.

(1999). *Contributions to philosophy.* Bloomington: Indiana University Press.

Helminski, K. (1992). *Living presence: A Sufi guide to mindfulness and the essential self.* New York: Tarcher/Perigree Books.

Hemenway, D., Vriniotis, M., & Miller, M. (2006). Is an armed society a polite society? Guns and road rage. *Accident Analysis and Prevention,* 38, 687–695.

Holt, R. R., & Silverstein, B. (Eds.). (1989). The image of the enemy: U.S. views of the Soviet Union [Special issue]. *Journal of Social Issues*, 45(2).

Horwitz, A. V. (2002). *Creating mental illness*. Chicago: University of Chicago Press.

Hsu, M. C., Schubiner, H., Lumley, M. A., Stracks, J. S., Clauw, D. J., & Williams, D. A. (2010). Sustained pain reduction through affective self-awareness in fibromyalgia: A randomized controlled trial. *Journal of General Internal Medicine*, 25, 1064–1070.

Hull, J. G. (1981). A self-awareness model of the causes and effects of alcohol consumption. *Journal of Abnormal Psychology*, 90, 586–600.

Human Security Report Project. (2007). *Human Security Brief 2007*. Vancouver, Canada: Human Security Report Project.

Huntington, Samuel P. (1996). *The Clash of Civilizations and the Remaking of the World Order*. New York: Simon & Schuster.

Husserl, E. (1999). *The idea of phenomenology*. Trans. L. Hardy. Dordrecht: Springer Netherlands. (Original work published 1907)

Institute of Medicine. (2011). *Relieving pain in America: A blueprint for transforming prevention, care, education, and research*. Washington, DC: National Academy of Sciences.

Jafari, M. T. (1995). *Mathnavi Ma'navi: A critical interpretation* (Vol. 4). Tehran, Iran: Alame Jafari.

(2004). *Dar Mahzare Hakim (In the presence of wisdom)*. Tehran, Iran: Alame Jafari.

James, W. (1958). *The varieties of religious experience: A study in human nature*. New York: New American Library.

(1971). A pluralistic universe. In R. B. Perry (Eds.), *Essays in radical empiricism and a pluralistic universe*. New York: Dutton.

Janov, A. (1970). *The primal scream. Primal therapy: The cure for neurosis*. New York: G. P. Putnam's Sons.

Jaspers, K. (1962). *Socrates, Buddha, Confucius, Jesus: The paradigmatic individuals*. New York: Harcourt, Brace.

Johnson, W., & Krueger, R. F. (2005). Higher perceived life control decreases genetic variance in physical health: Evidence from a national twin study. *Journal of Personality and Social Psychology*, 88, 165–73.

Johnson, D. E., Mueller, K. P., & Taft, W. H. (2002). *Conventional coercion across the spectrum of operations: The utility of U.S. military forces in the emerging environment*. Santa Monica, CA: RAND.

Jung, C. G. (1961). *Memories, dreams, reflections*. New York: Pantheon.

Jung, C. (1971). *Psychological types: Collected works*. Vol. 6. Trans. R. F. C. Hull. Bollingen Series XX. Princeton, NJ: Princeton University Press. (Originally published 1921)

(1966). *The spirit in man, art, and literature: Collected works*. Vol. 15. Trans. R. F. C. Hull. Bollingen Series XX. Princeton, NJ: Princeton University Press.

Jung, C. G., & Von Franz, M. L. (Eds.). (1964). *Man and his symbols*. New York: Dell.

Kabat-Zinn, J. (1990). *Full catastrophe living: Using the wisdom of your body and mind to face stress, pain, and illness.* New York: Random House.

(1994). *Wherever you go there you are.* New York: Hyperion Press.

(2003). Mindfulness-based interventions in context: Past, present, and future. *Clinical Psychology: Science and Practice,* 10, 144–156.

(2005). *Coming to our senses: Healing ourselves and the world through mindfulness.* New York: Hyperion Press.

Kadloubovsky, E., & Palmer, E. M. (Eds.). (1966). *The art of prayer: An orthodox anthology.* London: Faber and Faber.

Kanfer, F. H. (1970). Self-regulation: Research, issues, and speculations. In C. Neuringer & J. L. Michaels (Eds.), *Behavior modification in clinical psychology* (pp. 178–220). New York: Appleton-Century-Crofts.

Katz, C. (1992). All the world is staged: Intellectuals and the projects of ethnography. *Environment and Planning D: Society and Space,* 10, 495–510.

Keegan, J. (1993). *A history of warfare.* New York: Knopf.

Kelley, H. H., & Michela, J. L. (1980). Attribution theory and research. *Annual Review of Psychology,* 31, 457–501.

Kelman, H. C. (1965). *International behavior: A social-psychological analysis.* New York: Holt, Rinehart, & Winston.

Kierkegaard, S. (1959). *Either-or.* New York: Garden City.

(1989). *The sickness unto death: A Christian psychological exposition for edification and awakening.* New York: Penguin Books.

(1992). *Concluding unscientific postscript to philosophical fragments.* Trans. Howard & Edna Hong. Princeton, NJ: Princeton University Press.

(1998a). *The moment and late writings.* Trans. Howard & Edna Hong. Princeton, NJ: Princeton University Press.

(1998b). *The point of view.* Princeton, NJ: Princeton University Press.

Kohut, H. (1971). Peace Prize 1969: Laudation. *Journal of the American Psychoanalytic Association,* 19, 806–818.

Konijn, E. A., Nije Bijvank, M., & Bushman, B. J. (2007). I wish I were a warrior: The role of wishful identification in effects of violent video games on aggression in adolescent boys. *Developmental Psychology,* 43, 1038–1044.

Kross, E., Berman, M. G., Mischel, W., Smith, E. E., & Wager, T. D. (2011). Social rejection shares somatosensory representations with physical pain. *Proceedings of the National Academy of Sciences,* 108, 6270–6275.

Kruglanski, A. W., & Orehek, E. (2007). Partitioning the domain of social influence: Dual mode and system models and their alternatives. *Annual Review of Psychology,* 58, 291–316.

Kuhn, T. S. (1962). *The structure of scientific revolution.* Chicago: University of Chicago Press.

Kupperman, J. J. (2005). Morality, ethics, and wisdom. In R. Sternberg & J. Jordan (Eds.), *Handbook of mindfulness* (pp. 245–271). New York: Cambridge University Press.

Lachman, M. (2006). Perceived control over aging-related declines: Adaptive beliefs and behaviors. *Current Directions in Psychological Sciences,* 15, 282–286.

Lacina, B., & Gleditsch, N. P. (2005). Monitoring trends in global conflict: A new database in battle deaths. *European Journal of Population*, 21, 145–166.

Langer, E. J. (1975). The illusion of control. *Journal of Personality and Social Psychology*, 32, 311–328.

(1989). *Mindfulness*. Reading, MA: Addison-Wesley.

(1997). *The power of mindful learning*. Reading, MA: Addison-Wesley.

(2000). Mindful learning. *Current Directions in Psychological Science*, 9, 220–223.

(2005). *On becoming an artist: Reinventing yourself through mindful creativity*. New York: Ballantine Books.

(2009). *Counterclockwise: Mindful health and the power of possibility*. New York: Ballantine Books.

(2016). *The power of mindful learning*. Boston: De Capo Press.

Langer, E. J., & Abelson, R. P. (1974). A patient by any other name . . .: Clinician group difference in labeling bias. *Journal of Consulting and Clinical Psychology*, 42, 4–9.

Langer, E. J., Bashner, R., & Chanowitz, B. (1985). Decreasing prejudice by increasing discrimination. *Journal of Personality and Social Psychology*, 49, 113–120.

Langer, E. J., Blank, A., & Chanowitz, B. (1978). The mindlessness of ostensibly thoughtful action: The role of "placebic" information in interpersonal interaction. *Journal of Personality and Social Psychology*, 36, 635–42.

Langer, E. J., Carson, S., & Shih, M. (in press). Sit still and pay attention? *Journal of Adult Development*.

Langer E. J., & Rodin, J. (1976). The effects of choice and enhanced personal responsibility for the aged: A field experiment in an institutional setting. *Journal of Personality and Social Psychology*, 34, 191–198.

Lantieri, L., & Goleman, D. P. (2008). *Building emotional intelligence: Techniques to cultivate inner strength in children*. Boulder, CO: Sounds True.

Lausic, D., Tennebaum, G., Eccles, D., Jeong, A., & Johnson, T. (2009). Intrateam communication and performance in double tennis. *Research Quarterly for Exercise and Sport*, 80, 281–290.

Latour, B. (2004). How to talk about the body? The normative dimension of science studies. *Body and Society*, 10, 205–229.

LeDoux, J. (1996). *The emotional brain: The mysterious underpinnings of emotional life*. New York: Touchstone Books.

Lee, M. S., Pittler, M. H., & Ernst, E. (2007). External qigong for pain conditions: A systematic review of randomized clinical trials. *Journal of Pain*, 8, 827–831.

Lefkowitz, M. M., Huesmann, L. R., & Eron, L. D. (1978). Parental punishment: A longitudinal analysis of effects. *Archives of General Psychiatry*, 35, 186–191.

Li, R. (2020). The other essential pandemic office Trump eliminated. *Slate*, March 18. https://slate.com/technology/2020/03/coronavirus-social-behav ior-trump-white-house.html

Lieberman, M. D., Eisenberger, N. I., Crockett, M. J., Tom, S. M., Pfeifer, J. H., & Way, B. M. (2007). Putting feelings into words: Affect labeling disrupts amygdala activity in response to affective stimuli. *Psychological Science*, 18, 421–428.

Lifton, R. J. (2012). *Thought reform and the psychology of totalism*. Chapel Hill: University of North Carolina Press.

Lindorff, D. (2010). Your tax dollars at war: More than 53% of your tax payment goes to the military. *Common Dreams*, April 13. www.commondreams.org/views/2010/04/13/your-tax-dollars-war-more-53-your-tax-payment-goes-military

Linehan, M. M. (1993). *Skills training manual for treating borderline personality disorder*. New York: Guilford Press.

Linley, P. A., & Joseph, P. (2004). Toward a theoretical foundation for positive psychology in practice. In P. A. Linley & S. Joseph (Eds.), *Positive psychology in practice* (pp. 713–731). Hoboken, NJ: John Wiley & Sons.

Lipsey, M. W., Wilson, D. B., Cohen M. A., & Derzon, J. H. (1997). Is there a causal relationship between alcohol use and violence? A synthesis of the evidence. In M. Galanter (Ed.), *Recent developments in alcoholism: Vol. 13. Alcohol and violence: Epidemiology, neurobiology, psychology, and family issues*, (pp. 245–282). New York: Plenum Press.

Lopes, D. (2000). *Sensory deprivation*. Toronto, Canada: Coach House Books.

Lotringer, S. (Ed.). (1996). *Foucault live: Michael Foucault: Collected interviews, 1961–1984*. Trans. L. Hochroth & J. Johnson. New York: Semiotext(e).

Lowen, A. (1975). *Bioenergetics*. New York: Coward, McCann & Geoghegan.

Lumley, M. A., Cohen, J. L., Borszcz, G. S., Cano, A., Radcliffe, A., Porter, L., ... Keefe, F. J. (2011). Pain and emotion: A biopsychosocial review of recent research. *Journal of Clinical Psychology*, 67, 942–968.

Lykken, D., & Tellegen, A. (1996). Happiness is a stochastic phenomenon. *Psychological Science*, 7, 186–189.

Lyotard, J.-F. (1984). *The postmodern condition: A report on knowledge*. Trans. G. Bennington & B. Massumi. Minneapolis: University of Minnesota Press. (Original work published 1979)

MacAndrew, C., & Edgerton, R. (1969). *Drunken comportment: A social explanation*. Chicago: Aldine.

Maddux, J. E., Snyder, C. R., & Lopez, S. (2004). Towards a positive clinical psychology: Deconstructing the illness ideology and constructing an ideology of human strengths and potential. In P. A. Linley & S. Joseph (Eds.), *Positive psychology in practice* (pp. 320–334). Hoboken, NJ: John Wiley & Sons.

Malleson, A. (2002). *Whiplash and other useful illnesses*. Montreal, Canada: McGill-Queens University Press.

Marsella, A. J., & Higginbotham, H. (1984). Traditional Asian medicine: Applications to psychiatric services in developing nations. In P. Pedersen, N. Sartorius, & A. Marsella(Eds.), *Mental health services: The cross-cultural context* (pp. 175–198). Beverly Hills, CA: Sage.

Marsella, A. J., & Yamada, A. M. (2007). Culture and psychopathology: Foundations, issues, and directions. In S. Kitayama & D. Cohen (Eds.), *Handbook of cultural psychology* (pp. 787–818). New York: Guilford Press.

Martin, B. I., Deyo, R. A., Mirza, S. K., Turner, J. A., Comstock, B. A., Hollingworth, W., & Sullivan, S. D. (2008). Expenditures and health status among adults with back and neck problems. *Journal of the American Medical Association*, 299, 656–664.

Maultsby, M. C., Jr. (1971). Rational emotive imagery. *Rational Living*, 6, 24–27. (1975). *Help yourself to happiness*. New York: Institute for Rational Living.

Maultsby, M. C., Jr., & Ellis, A. (1974). *Technique for using rational emotive imagery*. New York: Institute for Rational Living.

May, R. (1975). *The courage to create*. New York: Norton.

McCrae, R. R., & Costa, P. T. (1990). *Personality in adulthood*. New York: Guilford Press.

McEvedy, C., & Jones, R. (1978). *Atlas of world population history*. London: A. Lane.

Medich, C., Stuart, E., & Chase, S. (1997). Healing through integration: Promoting wellness in cardiac rehabilitation. *Journal of Cardiovascular Nursing*, 11(3), 66–79.

Mega, M. S., Cummings, J. L., Salloway, S., & Malloy, P. (1997). *The limbic system in the neuropsychiatry of limbic and subcortical disorders*. Washington, DC: American Psychiatric Press.

Meichenbaum, D. (1977). *Cognitive behavior modification*. New York: Plenum Press.

Menec, V. H., Chipperfield, J. G., & Perry, R. P. (1999). Self-perceptions of health: A prospective analysis of mortality, control and health. *Journal of Gerontology: Psychological Sciences*, 54B, 85–93.

Merleau-Ponty, M. (1962). *Phenomenology of perception*. Trans. D. A. Landes. New York: Routledge. (Original work published 1945)

Merryfield, M. M. (2009). Moving the center of global education: From imperial world views that divide the world to double consciousness, contrapuntal pedagogy, hybridity, and cross-cultural competence. In J. L. Tucker (Eds.), *Visions in global education. The globalization of curriculum and pedagogy in teacher education and schools: Perspectives from Canada, Russia, and the United States* (pp. 219–223). New York: Peter Lang.

Mischkowski, D., Kross, E., & Bushman, B. J. (2012). Flies on the wall are less aggressive: Self-distanced reflection reduces angry feelings, aggressive thoughts, and aggressive behaviors. *Journal of Experimental Social Psychology*, 48, 1187–1191.

Mitra, S. (2008). Opioid-induced hyperalgesia: Pathophysiology and clinical implications. *Journal of Opioid Management*, 4, 23–130.

Moldoveanu, M., & Langer, E. (2002). When "stupid" is smarter than we are: Mindlessness and the attribution of stupidity. In R. J. Sternberg (Ed.), *Why smart people can be so stupid* (pp. 212–231). New Haven, CT: Yale University Press.

Molnar, D. S., Flett, G. L., Sadava, S. W., & Colautti, J. (2012). Perfectionism and health functioning in women with fibromyalgia. *Journal of Psychosomatic Research*, 73, 295–300.

Moreno, J. L. (1946). *Psychodrama* (Vol. 1). New York: Beacon House.

Nadeau, R. (1991). *Mind, machines and human consciousness.* Chicago: Contemporary Books.

Nagel, T. (2012). *Mind and cosmos: Why the materialist neo-Darwinian conception of nature is almost certainly false.* Oxford: Oxford University Press.

Nasr, S. H. (Ed.). (2007). *The essential Seyed Hossein Nasr.* Bloomington, IN: World Wisdom.

Nelson, G., & Prilleltensky, I. (2005). *Community psychology: In pursuit of liberation and wellbeing.* New York: Palgrave Macmillan.

Newberg, A., & Iversen, J. (2003). The neural basis of the complex mental task of meditation: Neurotransmitter and neurochemical considerations. *Medical Hypothesis*, 8, 282–291.

Noorani, A. (1980). *TalkheesolMohassal, known as NaqdeMohassal.* Tehran, Iran: University of Tehran-McGill.

Olweus, D. (1979). The stability of aggressive reaction patterns in males: A review. *Psychological Bulletin*, 86, 852–875.

Otis, J. (2007). *Managing chronic pain: A cognitive-behavioral therapy approach workbook.* Oxford: Oxford University Press.

Ovid. (n.d.). GigaQuotes. www.giga-usa.com/quotes/authors/ovid_a005.htm.

Pacini, R., & Epstein, S. (1999). The relation of rational and experiential information processing styles to personality, basic beliefs, and the ratio-bias phenomenon. *Journal of Personality and Social Psychology*, 76, 972–987.

Parker, I. (1989). *The crisis in modern social psychology, and how to end it.* London: Routledge.

Paul, L., & Weinert, C. (1999). Wellness profile of midlife women with a chronic illness. *Public Health Nursing*, 16, 341–350.

Paulhus, D. L., & Williams, K. M. (2002). The dark triad of personality: Narcissism, Machiavellianism, and psychopathy. *Journal of Research in Personality*, 36, 556–563.

Pearce, J. C. (2002). *The biology of transcendence: A blueprint of the human spirit.* Rochester, VT: Park Street Place.

Perls, F. S. (1969). *Gestalt therapy verbatim.* Moab, UT: Real People Press.

Perry, R. P. (2003). Perceived (academic) control and causal thinking in achievement settings. *Canadian Psychology*, 2, 35–49.

Perry, R. P., Hladkyj, S., Pekrun, R. H., & Pelletier, S. T. (2001). Academic control and action control in the achievement of college students: A longitudinal field study. *Journal of Educational Psychology*, 93, 776–789.

Peterson, C., Maier, S. F., & Seligman, M. E. P. (1995). *Learned helplessness: A theory for the age of personal control.* New York: Oxford University Press.

Petty, R. E., & Cacioppo, J. T. (1986a). *Communication and persuasion: Central and peripheral routes to attitude change.* New Yor: Springer-Verlag.

(1986b). The elaboration likelihood model of persuasion. In L. Berkowitz (Ed.), *Advances in experimental social psychology* (Vol. 19, pp. 123–205). San Diego, CA: Academic Press.

Pilisuk, M. (1982). Delivery of social support: The social inoculation. *American Journal of Orthopsychiatry*, 52, 20–31.

Pilisuk, M., McAllister, J., Rothman, J., & Larin, L. (2004). Social change, professionals and grassroots organizing. In M. Minkler (Ed.), *Community organizing and community building for health* (2nd ed., pp. 97–115). New Brunswick, NJ: Rutgers University Press.

Pilisuk, M., Minkler, M. (1980). Supportive networks: Life ties for the elderly. *Journal of Social Issues*, 36, 95–116.

Pilisuk, M., & Parks, S. H. (1986). *The healing web: Social networks and human survival*. Lebanon, NH: University Press of New England.

Pinker, S. (2011). *The better angels of our nature*. New York: Viking.

Pinxten, R. (2009). Universalism and relativism of knowledge dissipate: The intercultural perspective. In N. Note (Ed.), *Worldviews and cultures: Philosophical reflections from an intercultural perspective* (pp. 191–200). Berlin: Springer Verlag.

Polman, J., Orobio de Castro, B., & van Aken, M. (2008). Experimental study of the differential effects of playing versus watching violent video games on children's aggressive behavior. *Aggressive Behavior*, 34, 256–264.

Raimy, V. (1975). *Misunderstandings of the self*. San Francisco: Jossey-Bass.

Razee, S. (Ed.). (1993). *Najolbalaghe of Imam Alil (Alayhessalam)*. Qom, Iran: Hejrat.

Regehr, C., Cadell, S., & Jansen, K. (1999). Perceptions of control and long-term recovery from rape. *American Journal of Orthopsychiatry*, 69, 110–115.

Rehm, L. P. (1977). A self-control model of depression. *Behavior Therapy*, 8, 787–804.

Ricoeur, P. (1991). *A Ricoeur reader: Reflection and imagination*. Toronto, Canada: University of Toronto Press.

Richards, R. (Ed.). (2007). *Everyday creativity and new views of human nature: Psychological, social and spiritual perspectives*. Washington, DC: American Psychological Association.

Rimm, D. C., & Masters, J. C. (1979). *Behavior therapy* (Rev. ed.). New York: Academic Press.

Rodin, J. (1986). Aging and health: Effects of the sense of control. *Science*, 233, 1271–1276.

Rodin, J., & Langer, E. (1977). Long-term effects of a control-relevant intervention with the institutionalized aged. *Journal of Personality and Social Psychology*, 35, 897–902.

Rogers, C. (1961). *Becoming a person*. New York: Houghton Mifflin Harcourt.

Rotter, J. B. (1954). *Social learning and clinical psychology*. Englewood Cliffs, NJ: Prentice Hall.

Russell, B. (1903). A free man's worship. *The Independent Review* 1, 415–24. Available at https://users.drew.edu/~jlenz/br-fmw.pdf Repr.

Ruthig, J. C., Haynes, T. L., Stupnisky, R. H., & Perry, R. P. (2009). Perceived academic control: Mediating the effects of optimism and social support on college students' psychological health. *Social Psychology of Education*, 12, 233–249.

Sa'di, S. M. (1998). *Koleyyate Sa'di*. Tehran, Iran: Forooghi.

Sarason, S. (1988). *The psychological sense of community*. Cambridge, MA: Brookline Books.

Sardello, R. (2006). *Silence: The mystery of wholeness*. Benson, NC: Goldenstone Press.

Sarno, J. E. (1998). *The mindbody prescription: Healing the body, healing the pain*. New York: Warner Books.

Schmidt, S., Grossman, P., Schwarzer, B., Jena, S., Naumann, J., & Walach, H. (2011). Treating fibromyalgia with mindfulness-based stress reduction: Results from a 3-armed randomized controlled trial. *PAIN*, 152, 361–369.

Schneider, F. W., Gruman, J. A., & Coutts, L. M. (2012). *Applied social psychology: Understanding and addressing social and practical problems*. New York: Oxford University Press.

Schneider, K. (1998). Toward a science of the heart: Romanticism and the revival of psychology. *American Psychologist*, 53, 277–289.

(2011). Awakening to an awe-based psychology. *The Humanistic Psychologist*, 39, 247–252.

(2013). *The polarized mind: Why it's killing us and what we can do about it*. Colorado Springs, CO: University Professors Press.

(2018). The chief peril is not a DSM diagnosis but the polarized mind. *Journal of Humanistic Psychology*, 59, 99–106.

Schneider, K. & Fatemi, S. M. (2019). Polarized mind. *Scientific American*. https://blogs.scientificamerican.com/observations/todays-biggest-threat-the-polarizedmind/?previewid=FBAEF75B-F2E4-4D91-B88B353A4E17BD2F

Schubiner, H., & Betzold, M. (2012). *Unlearn your pain*. Pleasant Ridge, MI: Mind Body.

Schulz, R. (1976). Effects of control and predictability on the physical and psychological wellbeing of the institutionalized aged. *Journal of Personality and Social Psychology*, 33, 563–573.

Schulz, R., & Hanusa, B. H. (1978). Long-term effects of control and predictability enhancing interventions: Findings and ethical issues. *Journal of Personality and Social Psychology*, 36, 1194–1201.

Scileppi, J. A., Teed, E. L., & Torres, R. D. (2000). *Community psychology: A common sense approach to mental health*. Upper Saddle River, NJ: Prentice Hall.

Scruton, R. (2009). Confronting biology. In C. S. Titus (Ed.), *Philosophical psychology: Psychology, emotion and freedom* (pp. 68–107). Arlington, VA: Institute for the Psychological Sciences Press.

Segal, Z. V., Williams, J. M., & Teasdale, J. D. (2002). *Mindfulness-based cognitive therapy for depression: A new approach to preventing relapse*. New York: Guilford Press.

Seligman, M. E. P. (2002). *Authentic happiness: Using the new positive psychology to realize your potential for lasting fulfillment*. New York: Free Press.

Seligman, M. E. P., & Csikszentmihalyi, M. (Eds.). (2000). Positive psychology. *American Psychologist*, 55, 5–14.

Shariati, A. (1988). *Hajj*. Trans. Laleh Bakhtian. Tehran, Iran: Islamic Publications International.

Sherman, J. J., Turk, D. C., & Okifuji, A. (2000). Prevalence and impact of posttraumatic stress disorder-like symptoms on patients with fibromyalgia syndrome. *Clinical Journal of Pain*, 16, 127–134.

Shorter, E. (1993). *From paralysis to fatigue: A history of psychosomatic illness in the modern era*. New York: Free Press.

Silverman, S. M. (2009). Opioid-induced hyperalgesia: Clinical implications for the pain practitioner. *Pain Physician*, 12, 679–684.

Skinner, E. A. (1995). *Perceived control, motivation and coping*. Thousand Oaks, CA: Sage.

Smith, R. A., Wallston, B. S., Wallston, K. A., Forsberg, P. R., & King, J. E. (1984). Measuring desire for control of health care processes. *Journal of Personality and Social Psychology*, 47, 415–426.

Smyth, J. M., Stone, A. A., Hurewitz, A., & Kaell, A. (1999). Effects of writing about stressful experiences on symptom reduction in patients with asthma or rheumatoid arthritis: A randomized trial. *Journal of the American Medical Association*, 281, 1304–1309.

Solomon, J. L., Marshall, P., & Gardner, H. (2005). Crossing boundaries to generative wisdom. In R. Sternberg & J. Jordan (Eds.), *Handbook of mindfulness* (pp. 272–296). New York: Cambridge University Press.

Sorrentino, R. M. (2003). Motivated perception and the warm look: Current perspectives and future directions. In S. J. Spencer, S. Fein, M. P. Zanna, & J. M. Olson (Eds.), *Motivated social perception: The Ontario symposium* (Vol. 9, pp. 299–316). Mahwah, NJ: Erlbaum.

Sorrentino, R. M., & Higgins, E. T. (1986). Motivation and cognition: Warming to synergism. In R. M. Sorrentino & E. T. Higgins (Eds.), *The handbook of motivation and cognition: Foundations of social behavior* (pp. 3–19). New York: Guilford Press.

Spariosu, M. I. (2004). *Global intelligence and human development: Toward an ecology of global learning*. Cambridge, MA: MIT Press.

Spariosu, M. (2005). *Global intelligence and human development*. Cambridge, MA: MIT Press.

Sporer, S. L., Trinkl, B., & Guberova, E. (2007). Matching faces: Differences in processing speed of out-group faces by different groups. *Journal of Cross-Cultural Psychology*, 38, 398–412.

Steele, C. M., & Josephs, R. A. (1990). Alcohol myopia: Its prized and dangerous effects. *American Psychologist*, 45, 921–933.

Steinfeld, J. (1972). Statement in hearings before Subcommittee on Communications of Committee on Commerce (United States Senate, Serial #92–52) (pp. 25–27). Washington, DC: U.S. Government Printing Office.

Sternberg, R. (2005). *Handbook of mindfulness*. New York: Cambridge University Press.

Subra, B., Muller, D., Bègue, L., Bushman, B. J., & Delmas, F. (2010). Effects of alcohol and weapon cues on aggressive thoughts and behaviors. *Personality and Social Psychology Bulletin, 36*, 1052–1057.

Suh, E. M., Diener, E., & Fujita, F. (1996). Event and subjective well-being: Only recent events matter. *Journal of Personality and Social Psychology, 70*, 1091–1102.

Sundararajan, L. (2020). Hegemonic categorization of the other contributes to epistemological violence. *Theory & Psychology, 30*, 377–383.

Szyf, M., McGowan, P., & Meaney, M. J. (2008). The social environment and the epigenome. *Environmental and Molecular Mutagenesis, 49*, 146–160.

Tacey, D. (2006). *How to read Jung*. New York: Norton.

Taylor, K. (2004). *Brainwashing: The science of thought control*. Oxford: Oxford University Press.

Teasdale, J. D. (1999). Emotional processing, three modes of mind and the prevention of relapse in depression. *Behaviour Research and Therapy, 37* (Supplement 1), S53–S77.

Teasdale, J. D., & Chaskalson, M. (2011). How does mindfulness transform suffering? I: The nature of and origins of dukkha. *Contemporary Buddhism, 12*, 89–102.

ten Have-de Labije, J., & Neborsky, R. J. (2012). *Mastering intensive short-term dynamic psychotherapy: A roadmap to the unconscious*. London: Karnac Books.

Teo, T. (2005). *The critique of psychology: From Kant to postcolonial theory*. New York: Springer.

(2018). *Outline of theoretical psychology: Critical investigations*. London: Springer.

Tharoor, I. (2020). Coronavirus kills its first democracy. *Washington Post*, March 30. www.washingtonpost.com/world/2020/03/31/coronavirus-kills-its-first-democracy/

Thompson, J. K., & Heinberg, L. J. (1999). The media's influence on body image disturbance and eating disorders: We've reviled them, now can we rehabilitate them? *Journal of Social Issues, 55*, 339–353.

Thompson, S. C. (1981). Will it hurt less if I can control it? A complex answer to a simple question. *Psychological Bulletin, 90*, 89–101.

Ting, R. S.-K., & Sundararajan, L. (2018). *Culture, cognition, and emotion in China's religious ethnic minorities*. Palgrave Studies in Indigenous Psychology. https://doi.org/10.1007/978-3-319-66059-2_7

Topolski, D. (1989). *True blue: The story of the Oxford boat race mutiny*. London: Bantam Books.

Tremblay, R. E. (2000). The development of aggressive behavior during childhood: What have we learned in the past century? *International Journal of Behavioral Development, 24*, 129–141.

Turner, C. W., Layton, J. F., & Simons, L. S. (1975). Naturalistic studies of aggressive behavior: Aggressive stimuli, victim visibility, and horn honking. *Journal of Personality and Social Psychology, 31*, 1098–1107.

U.S. Census Bureau. (2010). International data base (IDB): Total midyear population for the world: 1950–2020. www.census.gov/ipc/wwww/idb/worldpop.php

U.S. Federal Bureau of Investigation. (2012). *Uniform crime reports*. Washington, DC: U.S. Government Printing Office.

Vaillant, G. (2008). *Spiritual evolution: A scientific defense of faith*. New York: Broadway Books.

VanderStoep, S. W., Fagerlin, A., & Feenstra, J. S. (2000). What do students remember from introductory psychology? *Teaching of Psychology*, 2, 89–92.

Wald, A. (n.d.). Treatment of irritable bowel syndrome in adults. www.uptodate.com/contents/treatment-of-irritable-bowel-syndrome-in-adults

Walitt, B., Fitzcharles, M. A., Hassett, A. L., Katz, R. S., Hauser, W., & Wolfe, F. (2011). The longitudinal outcome of fibromyalgia: A study of 1555 patients. *Journal of Rheumatology*, 38, 2238–2246.

Wallston, B. S., & Wallston, K. A. (1981). Health locus of control. In H. Lefcourt (Ed.), *Research with the locus of control construct* (Vol. I). New York: Academic Press.

Wallston, K. A., & Wallston, B. S. (1982). Who is responsible for your health? The construct of health locus of control. In G. Sanders & J. M. Suls (Eds.), *Social psychology of health and illness*. (pp. 65–95). Hillsdale, NJ: Erlbaum.

Walsh-Bowers, R. W. (2005). Expanding the terrain of constructing the subject. In M. C. Chung (Ed.), *Rediscovering the history of psychology: Essays inspired by the work of Kurt Danziger* (pp. 97–118). Dordrecht, Netherlands: Kluwer Academic.

Wang, C., Schmid, C. H., Rones, R., Kalish, R., Yinh, J., Goldenberg, D. L., ... McAlindon, T. (2010). A randomized trial of tai chi for fibromyalgia. *New England Journal of Medicine*, 363, 743–754.

Wessells, M. (1999). Culture, power, and community approaches to psychosocial assistance and healing. In K. Nader, N. Dubrow, & B. Stamm (Eds.), *Honoring differences: Cultural issues in the treatment of trauma and loss* (pp. 267–282). New York: Brunner Mazel.

Whitaker, R. (2010). *Anatomy of an epidemic: Magic bullets, psychiatric drugs, and the astonishing rise of mental illness in America*. New York: Broadway.

Wilkinson, R. G., & Pickett, K. (2009). *The spirit level*. New York: Bloomsbury Press.

Wilson, E. O. (1978). *On human nature*. Cambridge, MA: Harvard University Press.

(1998). *Consilience: The unity of knowledge*. London: Little, Brown.

Winnicott, D. W. (1965). *The maturational processes and the facilitating environment*. New York: Routledge.

(1971). *Playing and reality*. New York: Psychology Press.

(1975). *Through paediatrics to psycho-analysis: Collected papers*. New York: Brunner/Mazel.

Winston, A. (2001). Cause into function: Ernst Mach and the reconstruction of explanation in psychology. In C. D. Green, M. Shore, & T. Teo (Eds.), *The transformation of psychology: Influences of 19th-century philosophy, technology, and natural science* (pp. 107–131). Washington, DC: American Psychological Association.

Wittgenstein, L. (1968). *Philosophical investigations.* Trans. G. E. M. Anscombe (3rd ed.). Oxford: Basil Blackwell. (Original work published 1953)

Woolgar, S. (1988). *Science: The very idea.* Chichester, UK: Ellis Horwood.

York Al-Karam, C. (Ed.) (2018). *Islamically integrated psychotherapy: Uniting faith and professional practice* (pp. 275–291). West Conshohocken, PA: Templeton Press.

Yunus, M. B. (2007). Fibromyalgia and overlapping disorders: The unifying concept of central sensitivity syndromes. *Seminars in Arthritis and Rheumatism, 36,* 339–356.

Zajonc, R. B. (1984). On the primacy of affect. *American Psychologist, 39,* 117–123.

Zeidan, F., Martucci, K. T., Kraft, R. A., Gordon, N. S., McHaffie, J. G., & Coghill, R. C. (2011). Brain mechanisms supporting the modulation of pain by mindfulness meditation. *Journal of Neuroscience, 31,* 5540–5548.

Zenner, C., Herrnleben-Kurz, S., Walatch, H. (2014). Mindfulness-based interventions in schools: A systematic review and meta-analysis. *Frontiers in Psychology, 5,*603.

Ziegler, D. J. (2002). Freud, Rogers and Ellis: A comparative theoretical analysis. *Journal of Rational-Emotive & Cognitive-Behavior Therapy, 20,* 75–91.

Zoogman, S., Goldberg, S., Hoyt, W., & Miller, L. (2014). Mindfulness interventions with youth: A meta-analysis. *Mindfulness, 6,* 1–13.

Index

Lightning Source UK Ltd.
Milton Keynes UK
UKHW021958140621
385525UK00003B/15